Applied Anatomy & Physiology
for Manual Therapists

REVIEW GUIDE

Applied Anatomy & Physiology
for Manual Therapists

REVIEW GUIDE

Second Edition

Pat Archer

Lisa Nelson

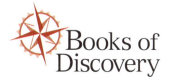

Second Edition

Copyright © 2021 Patricia A. Archer and Lisa A. Nelson
All rights reserved. No part of this book may be reproduced in any form, or by any electronic, mechanical or other means, without prior permission in writing from the publisher.

Published by Books of Discovery
Boulder, Colorado USA
booksofdiscovery.com
800.775.9227

ISBN: 978-0-9982663-7-4

Printed in the United States

15 14 13 12 11 10 9 8 7 6 5 4 3

Managing Editors: Alan Bernhard, Carrie Jenkins Williams
Designer: Jessica Xavier, Planet X Design

Disclaimer
Care has been taken to confirm the accuracy of the information presented in this publication and to describe generally accepted practices. However, the publisher, author, and editors are not responsible for omissions or errors or for any consequences from application of the information in this book, and make no warranty, expressed or implied, regarding the completeness or accuracy of the contents of this publication. Application of the information in a particular situation remains the practitioner's professional responsibility.

Contents

Learning Tips and Suggestions   vi

Unit I: Introduction to Anatomy, Physiology, and the Manual Therapies

Chapter 1: Applying Anatomy and Physiology to the Practice of Manual Therapy   1

Chapter 2: The Body and Its Terminology   16

Unit II: Cells, Tissues, and Membranes

Chapter 3: Chemistry, Cells, and Tissues   29

Chapter 4: Body Membranes and the Integumentary System   40

Unit III: Framework and Movement

Chapter 5: The Skeletal System   51

Chapter 6: The Skeletal Muscle System   64

Unit IV: Communication and Control

Chapter 7: The Nervous System   82

Chapter 8: Neuromuscular and Myofascial Connections   101

Chapter 9: The Endocrine System   113

Unit V: Circulation and Body Defense

Chapter 10: The Cardiovascular System   125

Chapter 11: The Lymphatic System   142

Chapter 12: Immunity and Healing   155

Unit VI: Metabolic Processes, Elimination, and Reproduction

Chapter 13: The Respiratory System   164

Chapter 14: The Digestive System   175

Chapter 15: The Urinary System   185

Chapter 16: The Reproductive System   194

Answer Key   203

Learning Tips and Suggestions

We all have preferences, habits, and opinions about the tools, resources, and methods that best support our learning. Many of us feel a need to walk, doodle, fidget, or talk to ourselves. Some of us like organized charts and exercises with one correct answer, while others prefer games or activities that allow us to explore lots of reference materials. Some people prefer the TV or stereo on, while others need quiet. We sometimes enjoy working in a group and at other times simply need space to review by ourselves. The important thing is to identify what works for *you*.

This *Review Guide* was written to provide you (the student) with learning tools, ideas, and options. It includes a variety of exercises to help you organize, experience, think about, and connect to the essential A&P details and concepts of *Applied Anatomy and Physiology for Manual Therapists*. While some activities are simply blank illustrations from the textbook to help you review or quiz your recall, other exercises provide new and different ways of looking at the information to deepen your understanding. For example, the crossword puzzles and fill-in exercises will help you focus on the simple declarative information such as names, locations, and definitions. Other activities like model building and coloring provide more active kinesthetic learning opportunities, while charting and mind mapping exercises can help you visually and mentally organize the information in several different ways.

Whether you decide to work through every exercise in order, jump around, or pick and choose just a few exercises from a chapter, here are some tips and suggestions to help you maximize your review time.

- **Use the key topics table** at the beginning of each chapter to identify and choose specific learning exercises that cover the information you want to review.
- **Use the chapter quizzes** either first to help you identify the topics you need to review the most, or last to test your knowledge and comprehension.
- **Try different types of exercises** to help you identify the ones that work best for you as well as the ones that challenge your mind to look at the information in different ways. Remember, methods that are comfortable and familiar generally make it easier for us to grasp facts. But activities that are less comfortable often help us develop deeper understandings.
- **Note activities you like** that are introduced in the first few chapters and adapt them to the content in other chapters. Several examples of these adaptable exercises include:
  - Charts and tables
  - Mind maps, Venn diagrams, and other graphic organizers
  - Concept maps
  - Flash cards (including several creative ways to make and use them)
  - Mnemonics
  - Analogies, stories, and poems

Finally, if you are looking for more exercises, study tips, or resources, please visit the Books of Discovery website. Be sure to click on the link for the TIPP™ Learning Assessment if you are interested in insights about your personal learning process.

Happy studying!
Lisa & Pat

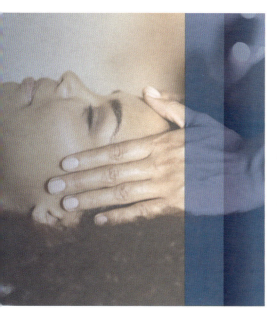

1

Applying Anatomy and Physiology to the Practice of Manual Therapy

Use this list to choose learning exercises that will help you expand and solidify your understanding of key topics. To test your knowledge, try the Review Quiz at the end of the chapter.

Key Topics	Exercise
• Terminology	1
• Levels of Body Organization	2–4
• Homeostasis and Feedback Mechanisms	4–7
• Categories and Common Names for Different Manual Therapies	9
• Benefits and Physiologic Effects of Manual Therapy	8–10
• Body Systems: Primary Components and General Functions	10–12

EXERCISE 1 • Terminology Crossword

Use this crossword to review and test your ability to define key terms from Chapter 1.

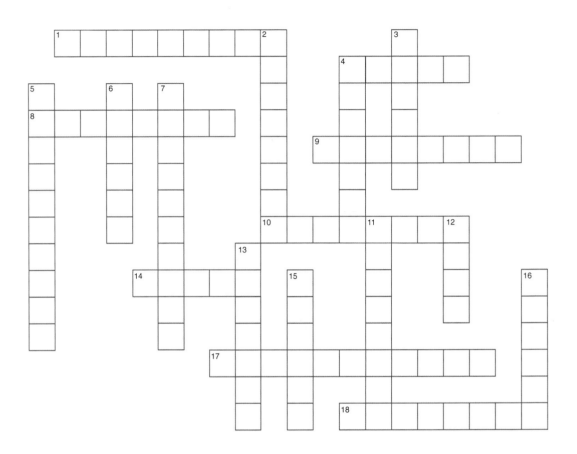

ACROSS

1. Sense organs sensitive to specific types of stimuli.
4. Can serve as the integration center in a feedback loop.
8. This health and wellness approach is guided by the principle that the physical body, cognitive processes (mind), and emotional or spiritual aspect are inseparable parts of a whole and integrated person.
9. The most common homeostatic feedback loop.
10. These regional or body-wide manual therapy effects are mediated by cellular, circulatory, and/or nervous system functions.
14. Group of tissues working together to accomplish specific tasks.
17. A level of internal stability or balance.
18. A living thing that functions as a whole.

DOWN

2. Any internal or external change in the environment.
3. Patterned and purposeful application of touch and/or movement with therapeutic intent is called _____ therapy.
4. A positive change in health or well-being caused by manual therapy regardless of the particular form utilized.
5. Study of the body's functional processes.
6. Group of like cells working together.
7. Manual therapy effects that create physical changes such as stretching or loosening.
11. Target cell, tissue, or organ that responds to a specific stimulus.
12. Basic functional unit of the body.
13. The form and structure of an organism.
15. A specific and measurable change due to a particular manual therapy technique.
16. Group of organs working together to accomplish a specific set of tasks.

EXERCISE 2 • Describing the Levels of Organization

Fill in the appropriate labels for the six different levels of body organization and provide a definition for each. If you need to refresh your memory, refer to Figure 1.1 in your text.

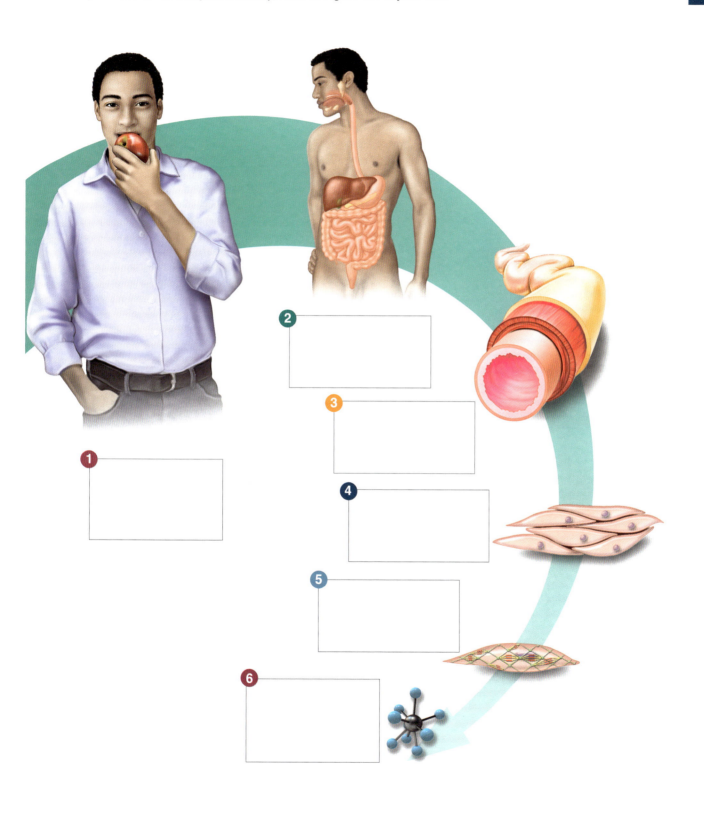

EXERCISE 3 • Describing the Levels of Organization

Draw diagrams for the five levels of body organization described in 2–6 below. If you need to refresh your memory, refer to Figure 1.1 in your text.

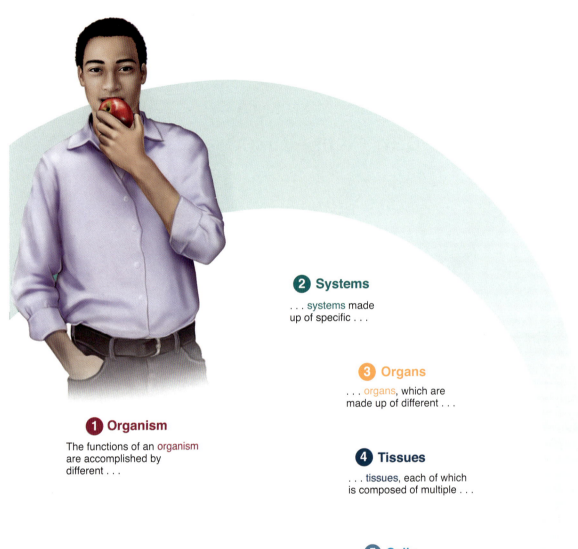

2 Systems

... systems made up of specific ...

3 Organs

... organs, which are made up of different ...

1 Organism

The functions of an organism are accomplished by different ...

4 Tissues

... tissues, each of which is composed of multiple ...

5 Cells

... cells composed of many different ...

6 Chemicals

... atoms and molecules.

EXERCISE 4 • Mnemonics

Mnemonics are helpful memory cues for recalling lists of information. To create a mnemonic, identify the first letter of each word in the list you want to remember. Next, come up with a memorable saying by stringing together words that utilize the same first letters (silly or suggestive themes seem to work best). The following mnemonic is an example created for recalling the levels of body organization.

Body = **B**odies
System = **S**ensing
Organ = **O**rganized
Tissue = **T**ouch
Cell = **C**onstantly
Chemical = **C**hange

Use the spaces provided below to come up with mnemonics for the parts of a homeostatic feedback mechanism and the seven categories of manual therapy.

Parts of a Homeostatic Mechanism

Stimulus—**S** _____

Receptor—**R** _____

Integration center—**I** _____

Effector—**E** _____

Categories of Manual Therapy

Swedish—**S** _____

Myofascial—**M** _____

Neuromuscular—**N** _____

Lymphatic—**L** _____

Movement therapies—**M** _____

Reflexive/zone therapies—**R** _____

Energy techniques—**E** _____

1: Applying Anatomy and Physiology to the Practice of Manual Therapy

EXERCISE 5 • Homeostasis Flow Chart

Define the four components of a homeostatic feedback loop. Next, complete the flow chart by placing each component in its correct position. Refer to Figure 1.2 in the text if you need to refresh your memory.

1. Integration center _____

2. Stimulus _____

3. Effector _____

4. Receptor _____

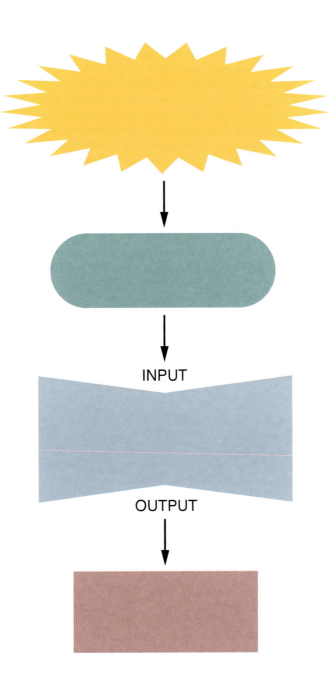

EXERCISE 6 • Negative and Positive Feedback

Homeostatic mechanisms are either negative or positive feedback loops. In a negative feedback loop, the response of the effector **1.** _____ the original stimulus, while in a positive feedback loop, the effector's response **2.** _____ the original stimulus.

Copy your answers for 1 and 2 into the corresponding boxes in the diagrams below. Then, color and label the rest to complete the diagrams for negative and positive feedback. Refer to Figure 1.3 if you need to review.

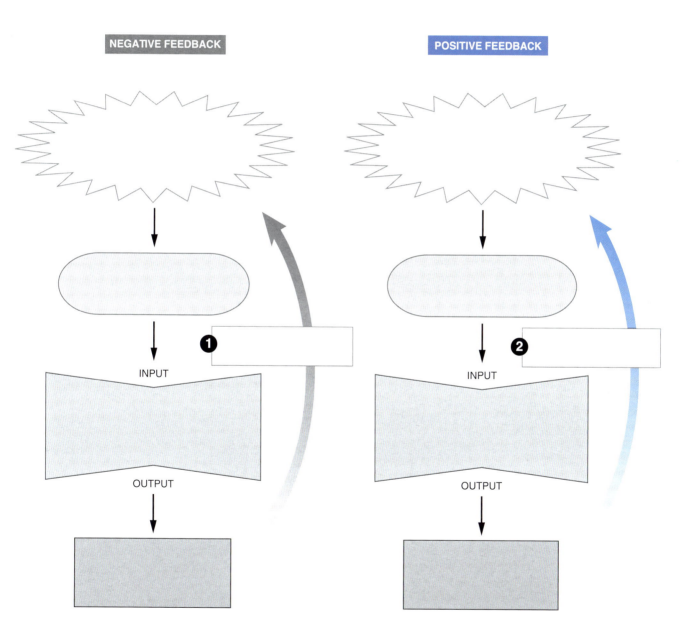

1: Applying Anatomy and Physiology to the Practice of Manual Therapy

EXERCISE 7 • Linking Body, Mind, and Spirit

From a holistic perspective, the definition of homeostasis can be broadened to include the balance or dynamic equilibrium that exists between body, mind, and spirit.

Explore this concept by writing down how the status of your body, mind, or spirit can affect the other aspects of this holistic balance. There are many correct answers for each graphic organizer. The answer key provides one example of each. Compare your answers with those of your classmates.

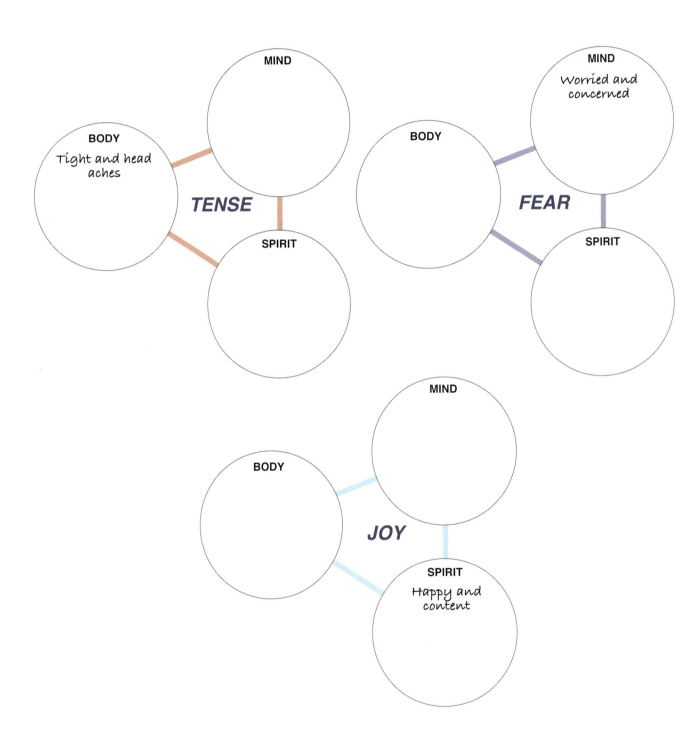

EXERCISE 8 • Benefits and Effects of Manual Therapy

*Identify each of the following as either a benefit (**B**) or physiologic effect (**E**) of manual therapy.*

1. _____ Enhanced sense of well-being

2. _____ Releasing adhered connective tissue

3. _____ Reduction of edema

4. _____ Decreased anxiety/stress

5. _____ Decreased pain

6. _____ Improved mental focus

7. _____ Improved sleep patterns

8. _____ Loosening or softening muscles and/or connective tissue

9. _____ Unwinding muscles and connective tissue

10. _____ Improved local venous flow

Think of some physiological effects of manual therapies. Use the columns below to list and identify those effects as either structural or systemic.

Structural Effect   **Systemic Effect**

EXERCISE 9 • Manual Therapy Categories

Fill in the blanks in the table below. Refer to Table 1.1 in the text if you need to refresh your memory.

CATEGORY	DESCRIPTION	PRIMARY THERAPEUTIC INTENTION	COMMON NAMES
Swedish or relaxation	**1.**	• Relaxation • Stress and anxiety reduction • Reconnecting • Grounding	**2.** Relaxation massage, or . . . • •
Myofascial	**3.** Any technique focused on: • • • fascia and other connective tissues Usually done with no lubricant or with minimal amounts of lubricant	**4.** Improve structural alignment, plus . . . • •	**5.** Aston-Patterning®, Craniosacral therapy, and . . . • • •
6.	Any technique that reduces resting muscle tension	**7.** Balance muscle tension, plus . . . • •	**8.** Active Release Techniques® (ART), Muscle Energy Technique (MET), and . . . • • •
Lymphatic	Any system of light to moderate-depth strokes based on A&P of the lymphatic system	**9.** Stimulate: • • •	• Complete decongestive therapy (CDT) • Lymphatic facilitation • Lymphatic massage • Lymphedema techniques • Manual Lymphatic Drainage (MLD)
10.	Focused, patterned, conscious movement and/or positioning	**11.** Achieve pain-free movement, plus . . . • • •	• Alexander Technique • Feldenkrais Method® • Hakomi Method • Qigong • Rosen Method • Tai chi • Trager® Approach
Reflexive/zone therapies	**12.**	• Improve systemic and organ functions • Decrease pain • Enhance general well-being and energy flow	**13.** Acupressure, Acupuncture, and . . . • • •
14.	Touching/holding/stroking (with or without physical contact) of chakras, energy zones, or chi points	**15.** Decongest, balance, or improve activity of energy also known as chi, or . . . • •	**16.** Aura techniques, Ayurvedic techniques, and . . . • •

EXERCISE 10 • Creating a Body Systems Table

Condensing information and organizing it in a table can make it easier to access and learn. Use the figures at the end of Chapter 1 and your own resources to create a quick reference for the systems of the body, their components, functions, and manual therapy connections. Some items have been filled in for you to get you started and the answer key offers possible responses.

BODY SYSTEM	COMPONENTS	FUNCTIONS	MANUAL THERAPY LINKS
Integumentary	Skin and its glands Hair Nails Sensory receptors	1.	Therapeutic interface for touch therapies
Skeletal	2.	Structure Protects vital organs Levers for muscles Blood cell production Mineral storage	3.
Muscular	4.	5.	Structural effects due to changes in muscles
Nervous	6.	Communication Coordination Control	7.
Endocrine	8.	Communication Coordination Control	9.
Cardiovascular	Blood Heart Blood vessels	10.	11.
Lymphatic/ immune	12.	13.	Specialty techniques boost fluid return and enhanced well-being improves immune function
Respiratory	Nose, sinuses, pharynx, larynx, trachea, bronchi, lungs	14.	15.
Digestive	16.	17.	Zone therapies target specific organs to improve function
Urinary	18.	Cleanses the blood Elimination of liquid wastes Regulation of pH, fluid, and electrolyte balances	Little direct effect except from zone therapies and lymphatic techniques
Reproductive	19.	Reproduction	20.

1: Applying Anatomy and Physiology to the Practice of Manual Therapy

EXERCISE 11 • Body Systems Anatomy Mind Map

Instead of a table, a mind map is an alternative way to organize information. Like a table, it condenses the information, but the map organizes it spatially instead of linearly.

Use the mind map below to identify the structural components of each body system. One system has been done for you to get you started and the answer key offers possible responses.

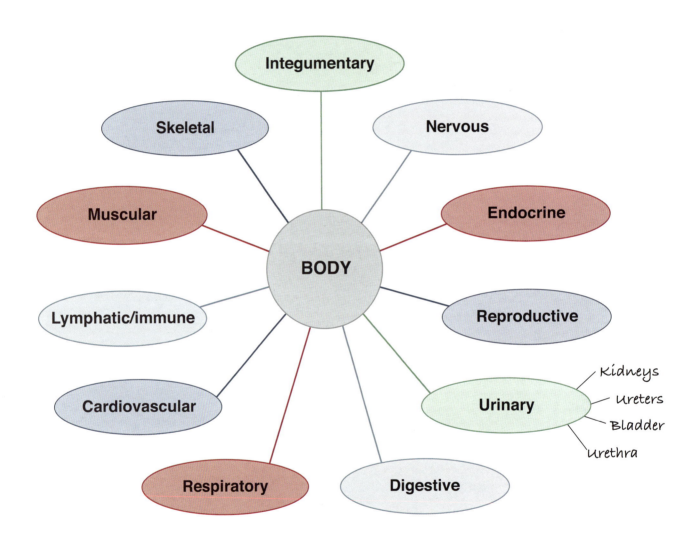

REVIEW GUIDE

EXERCISE 12 • Body Systems Physiology Mind Map

Use this mind map to note each system's functions. Again, one system is done for you to help get you started and the answer key offers possible responses. In addition, add colors to group systems together according to their common functions: covering; framework and movement; communication and control; circulation and body defense; metabolic processes and elimination; reproduction.

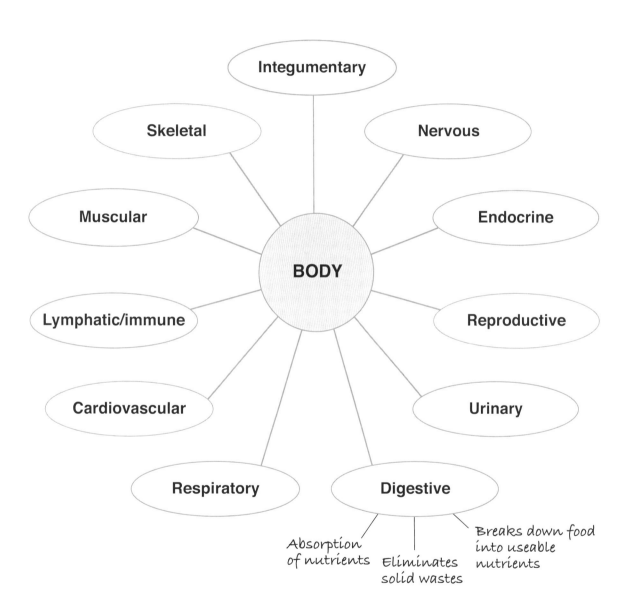

REVIEW QUIZ

Applying Anatomy and Physiology to the Practice of Manual Therapy

Multiple Choice: Select the one best answer.

1. A group of cells working to perform a common function is called what?
   A. tissue
   B. membrane
   C. organ
   D. tumor

2. A system is a group of _____ working to perform a set of common functions.
   A. tissues
   B. cells
   C. organs
   D. cells and tissue

3. Any change in the internal or external environment is called
   A. metabolism.
   B. stimulus.
   C. cellular shift.
   D. homeostasis.

4. What type of feedback is it when the response counteracts the original stimulus?
   A. positive
   B. negative
   C. metabolic
   D. simple

5. Which statement below is the best definition of homeostasis?
   A. shifting the metabolism to match changing energy demands
   B. maintaining the status of a specific system
   C. a dynamic equilibrium between physiologic processes needed to sustain life
   D. sharing the physiologic demands for nutrition and waste removal between all body systems

6. Which of the following is a primary component of the urinary system?
   A. pancreas
   B. kidney
   C. liver
   D. gallbladder

7. The spleen is a primary component of which body system?
   A. digestive
   B. urinary
   C. lymphatic
   D. endocrine

8. The pancreas is a key organ in which two systems?
   A. endocrine and digestive
   B. urinary and cardiovascular
   C. digestive and respiratory
   D. endocrine and lymphatic

9. The primary organs of the cardiovascular system are _____ and _____.
   A. spleen; blood vessels
   B. neurons; nephrons
   C. lymph nodes; vessels
   D. blood vessels; heart

10. Which of the following would be classified as a movement therapy?
    A. Aston-Patterning®
    B. wellness massage
    C. Feldenkrais Method®
    D. Active Release Techniques®

11. Which category of manual therapy is defined as any form with the intention to stretch, loosen, or broaden fascia and other connective tissues?
    A. Swedish/relaxation massage
    B. myofascial/deep tissue
    C. neuromuscular
    D. reflexive/zone therapy

12. Which category of manual therapy applies light or deep pressure to stimulate defined energy zones, dermatomes, or points on the body?
    A. Swedish/relaxation massage
    B. myofascial/deep tissue
    C. neuromuscular
    D. reflexive/zone therapy

13. Reduction of stress and improved mental focus are examples of
   A. structural effects.
   B. systemic effects.
   C. placebo effects.
   D. benefits of manual therapy.

14. Reduction of pain and improved range of motion are examples of
   A. benefits of all manual therapy.
   B. neuromuscular benefits.
   C. physiologic effects.
   D. structural effects.

15. The primary intentions of the movement therapies category of manual therapy include facilitating pain-free range of movement and
   A. releasing holding patterns.
   B. increasing circulation.
   C. improving posture.
   D. stimulating edema uptake.

16. Which of the following is an example of a structural effect of manual therapy?
   A. stretching muscles
   B. improved sleep patterns
   C. reduction of pain
   D. reduction of edema

17. Which category of manual therapy applies sliding and gliding techniques with a lubricant to create relaxation and reduce stress?
   A. energy
   B. Swedish
   C. myofascial
   D. zone/reflexive

18. Which of these manual therapy styles would be classified as reflexive/zone therapy?
   A. Hakomi
   B. NeuroKinetic Therapy®
   C. spa massage
   D. shiatsu

19. The primary intentions of reflexive/zone therapies include decreasing pain, improving systemic and organ functions, and
   A. enhancing general well-being.
   B. helping to release emotional holding patterns.
   C. improving structural alignment.
   D. balancing skeletal muscle tension.

20. What system has the primary function of returning fluid and protein to blood?
   A. cardiovascular
   B. immune
   C. lymphatic
   D. urinary

21. The primary functions of the urinary system include
   A. helping to balance fluids and blood pH.
   B. returning 100% of fluid from capillary filtrate to blood.
   C. transporting nutrients and waste.
   D. maintaining venous and arterial volumes.

22. What system is responsible for carrying out oxygen and carbon dioxide exchange for the body?
   A. digestive
   B. endocrine
   C. respiratory
   D. urinary

23. Which body system is responsible for creating movement?
   A. skeletal
   B. nervous
   C. endocrine
   D. muscular

24. Functions of the skeletal system include providing the structural framework for the body, protecting vital organs, and
   A. creating movement.
   B. serving as the site of blood cell production.
   C. breaking down of vitamins and minerals.
   D. serving as a primary storage site for energy.

25. The primary components of the integumentary system include skin, hair, nails, and
   A. sensory receptors.
   B. blood vessels.
   C. sinuses.
   D. nodes.

1: Applying Anatomy and Physiology to the Practice of Manual Therapy   15

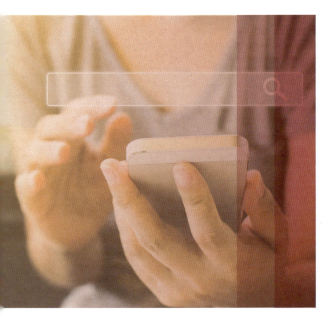

2

The Body and Its Terminology

Use this list to choose learning exercises that will help you expand and solidify your understanding of key topics. To test your knowledge, try the Review Quiz at the end of the chapter.

Key Topics	Exercise
• Terminology and Word Parts	1, 4, 10
• Body Planes	2
• Location and Movement Terms	3
• Body Cavities	5
• Body Regions	6 & 7
• Pathology Terms and Disease Classification	8 & 9

EXERCISE 1 • Flash Cards

Flash cards are a common study tool, especially for learning new terms and other straightforward declarative facts. For example, a flash card can have a new term on one side and its definition on the other, or a body system on one side and its components on the other. Whether you use an online tool such as cram.com or index cards, flash cards help you study in two ways: (1) making flash cards requires you to collect and organize new information and (2) the finished product is a portable study and review tool. The cards can be used while commuting via public transportation, waiting in line at the bank, or during a quick coffee break. You can use them to quiz study partners or organize them to help you keep track of which information you are sure of and what you need to continue to work on.

Here are a few variations on flash cards:

- **Color**—Consider using different colors for your cards or writing to categorize or organize flash cards. For example, in this chapter, you are learning terms for movement, location, body cavities, and body regions. Consider making each category of term a different color. This will help you determine which particular terms you need to focus your review and study on as well as which categories of terms are the most challenging for you.

- **Diagrams and sticky notes**—If you like to think in pictures instead of words, you may want to use blank body diagrams and sticky notes instead of flash cards. Print terms on the notes and simply stick the words to the appropriate body region on the blank diagram. If you need to learn verbal definitions, print a chart that has all the definitions on it. Then use the same "sticky words" and match the correct term with the definition.

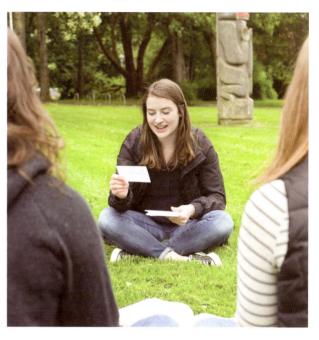

- **Audio "flash cards"**—If you spend long hours commuting in your car, reviewing information in an auditory manner with auditory flash cards could be a good option. To create these flash cards, simply use your favorite recording app on your phone or computer. Have a list of terms and definitions you want to review and make a recording that has pauses in it for you to repeat terms and/or define them. For example, you could record the word "gluteal" and then leave a space to repeat the term. Next record "Gluteal means" and leave a pause of 5 to 10 seconds before saying, "Gluteal means buttocks." When you play the recording back, you will notice you have a space to repeat the term to help you practice the correct pronunciation as well as a space to define the term before the definition is given to you. This is similar to the way many people learn a foreign language.

EXERCISE 2 • Planes of the Body

Label each of the planes and cross sections of the body. Use Figure 2.2 in your text if you need to refresh your memory.

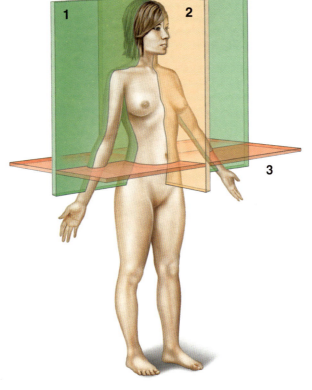
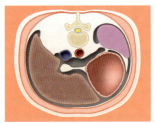
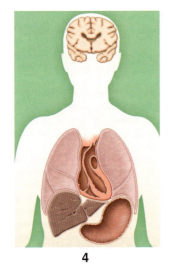
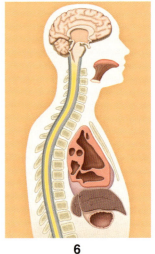

1. _____ plane
2. _____ plane
3. _____ plane
4. _____ section
5. _____ section
6. _____ section

EXERCISE 3 • Location and Movement Terms Crossword

Use this crossword to review and test your ability to define the location and movement terms from Chapter 2.

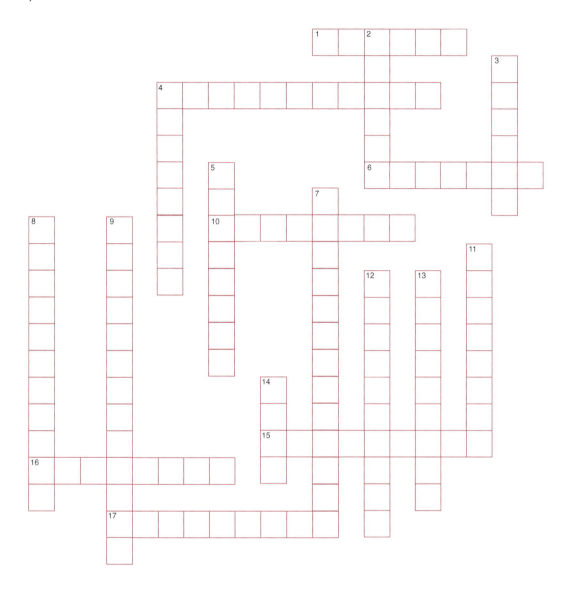

ACROSS

1. The sternum is _____ to the pectoral region.
4. On the same side of the median.
6. Farther from the midline.
10. Closer to the point of attachment.
15. Increasing the joint angle.
16. Front.
17. Moving away from the midline in the frontal plane.

DOWN

2. Another term for posterior.
3. The foot is _____ to the knee.
4. Below; caudal.
5. Another term for superior.
7. Multi-planar motion around a single point.
8. The scalp is _____ to the skull.
9. The eyes are _____ to one another.
11. Pivot around a single axis.
12. AB- or adduction in the transverse plane is referred to as _____.
13. The opposite of ABduction.
14. The bones are _____ to the skin.

EXERCISE 4 • Mix-and-Match Word Parts

Match the words in column A to their best definition from column B. Some of these words are made-up terms that you should be able to match by knowing the meaning of the prefix, suffix, and/or word root.

Column A

_____ **1.** Unicycle

_____ **2.** Contradictions

_____ **3.** Myositis

_____ **4.** Interosseous membrane

_____ **5.** Pseudonym

_____ **6.** Tulipoma

_____ **7.** Hemisphere

_____ **8.** Malcontent

_____ **9.** Retropatellar

_____ **10.** Antechamber

Column B

A. False name

B. One with poor socialization

C. One-wheeled cycle

D. Opposing thoughts or ideas

E. Entry hall or room

F. Behind the kneecap

G. A membrane between two bones

H. Inflamed muscle tissue

I. Tumor on a cup-shaped flower

J. One half of a round object

Now that you get the idea, have some fun using the terms in Table 2.3 of the text to make up some of your own words and matching definitions.

EXERCISE 5 • Body Cavities Color and Label

Color the ventral cavities one color and the dorsal cavities another. Next, label each of the individual cavities. If you need to refresh your memory, refer to Figure 2.11 in your text.

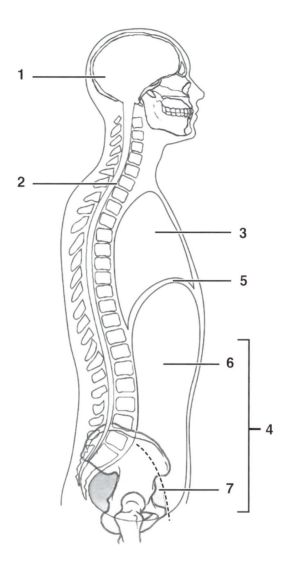

1. _____
2. _____
3. _____
4. _____
5. _____
6. _____
7. _____

EXERCISE 6 • Body Regions Matching

Match the name of the body region with the proper description.

_____ **1.** Fibular

_____ **2.** Crural

_____ **3.** Olecranal

_____ **4.** Coxal

_____ **5.** Cephalic

_____ **6.** Thoracic

_____ **7.** Pedal

_____ **8.** Sural

_____ **9.** Temporal

_____ **10.** Volar

_____ **11.** Carpal

_____ **12.** Occipital

_____ **13.** Gluteal

_____ **14.** Inguinal

_____ **15.** Lumbar

_____ **16.** Nasal

_____ **17.** Femoral

_____ **18.** Axillary

_____ **19.** Pectoral

_____ **20.** Popliteal

A. Foot

B. Head or cranium

C. Groin

D. Lower leg

E. Side of head

F. Back of hand

G. Posterior elbow

H. Wrist

I. Nose

J. Lateral side of leg

K. Lateral hip

L. Thigh; upper leg

M. Rib cage

N. Calf of leg

O. Armpit

P. Anterior upper chest

Q. Posterior head

R. Posterior knee

S. Low back

T. Buttocks

EXERCISE 7 • Body Regions Labeling

Label all of the body regions asked for on the diagram. If you need to refresh your memory, refer to Figures 2.8 through 2.10 in your text.

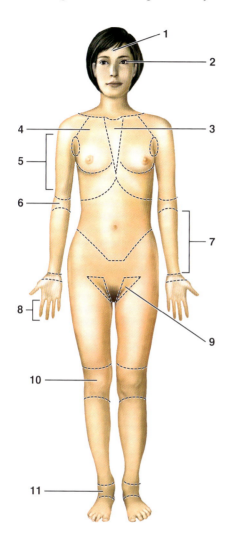
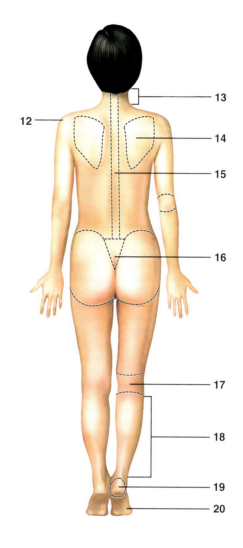

1. _____
2. _____
3. _____
4. _____
5. _____
6. _____
7. _____
8. _____
9. _____
10. _____
11. _____
12. _____
13. _____
14. _____
15. _____
16. _____
17. _____
18. _____
19. _____
20. _____

2: The Body and Its Terminology

EXERCISE 8 • Pathology Terms Case Report

To review the pathology terms, answer the following questions using the case report below.

John Jones goes to his doctor with a sore throat and headache. He explains that he has been feeling tired and generally run-down for a few days, but yesterday he woke up with a severe sore throat that feels scratchy and swollen, and it hurts to swallow. He didn't sleep well last night and thinks he has a fever as well. The doctor's examination finds swollen lymph nodes in his neck, a fever of 102°F, and red and pus-marked tonsils. He tells John that he has tonsillitis and that he needs to have his tonsils removed as soon as possible. The doctor believes John will recover completely within 2 or 3 days after surgery with a prescription of antibiotics.

1. What is the etiology? _____

_____

2. What is the diagnosis? _____

_____

3. What are the symptoms? _____

_____

4. What are the signs? _____

_____

5. What is the prognosis? _____

_____

Now try writing your own mini case report including the elements 1–5 as listed above.

EXERCISE 9 • Classes of Disease Table

Fill in the spaces in the table below that lists the six major classifications of disease, their definitions, and examples of each.

DISEASE CLASSIFICATION	DESCRIPTION	EXAMPLES
INFECTIOUS	1.	2.
3.	4.	Allergies Mesothelioma Asbestosis
5.	Disease caused by a particular genetic trait or flaw passed from one generation to the next	6.
NUTRITIONAL & LIFESTYLE	7.	8.
9.	10.	Lupus Rheumatoid arthritis Multiple sclerosis
11.	Caused by abnormal cells that divide uncontrollably and may invade surrounding tissues or other body systems	12.

EXERCISE 10 • A&P Terminology Crossword

Use this crossword to review and test your ability to define a variety of terms from Chapter 2.

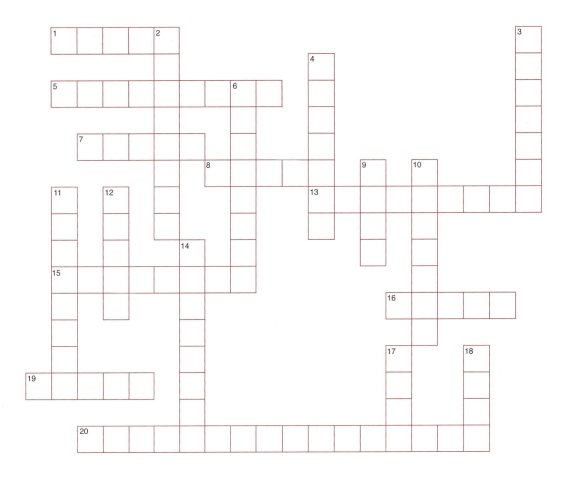

ACROSS

1. Sudden or rapid onset.
5. Posterior knee.
7. Tarsal region.
8. The term arthritis means inflammation of a _____ (refer to your word parts).
13. Posterior elbow.
15. Neck region.
16. The prefix pseudo means _____.
19. A bone-breaking cell could be called an osteo_____ (refer to your word parts).
20. A sign or symptom that could be made worse by a particular course of treatment.

DOWN

2. The cause of a disease.
3. Forehead region.
4. A subjective indicator of disease.
6. Point of the shoulder.
9. To describe a layer around something else, the prefix _____ can be used.
10. Chronic diseases and conditions have a _____ or long-term onset.
11. Upper arm region.
12. Fluid found within a cell can be called _____ cellular fluid (refer to your word parts).
14. Area of the shoulder blade.
17. Pedal region.
18. A fever is a _____ of disease because it is measurable.

26 REVIEW GUIDE

REVIEW QUIZ

The Body and Its Terminology

Multiple Choice: Select the one best answer.

1. What is the name of the plane that divides the body into front and back regions?
   A. sagittal/median
   B. frontal/coronal
   C. horizontal/transverse
   D. posterior/dorsal

2. What plane divides the body into right and left sides?
   A. sagittal/median
   B. frontal/coronal
   C. horizontal/transverse
   D. posterior/dorsal

3. The two ventral cavities are _____ and _____.
   A. abdominal and pelvic
   B. cranial and sacral
   C. abdominal and cranial
   D. thoracic and abdominopelvic

4. What terms are used to describe the location of a structure in relationship to the midline of the body?
   A. anterior, posterior
   B. proximal, distal
   C. dorsal, ventral
   D. medial, lateral

5. The directional term superior is used to describe a structure as being
   A. on the opposite side of the body.
   B. closer to the head.
   C. closer to the point of attachment of an extremity to the trunk.
   D. closer to the body surface.

6. What term describes the position of two points that are on opposite sides of the midline?
   A. contralateral
   B. ipsilateral
   C. medial
   D. distal

7. The elbow can be described as being _____ to the wrist.
   A. superior
   B. posterior
   C. proximal
   D. inferior

8. What is the anatomic term for the region of the head?
   A. cranial
   B. cervical
   C. caudal
   D. occipital

9. The posterior aspect of the knee is called the _____ region.
   A. sural
   B. femoral
   C. crural
   D. popliteal

10. What is the anatomic term for the armpit?
    A. acromion
    B. axilla
    C. humeral
    D. olecranal

11. The inguinal body region is more commonly known as the
    A. groin.
    B. buttocks.
    C. hip.
    D. chest.

12. An anterior movement along the sagittal plane that decreases the angle between two bones is called
    A. extension.
    B. ABduction.
    C. flexion.
    D. adduction.

13. Movement about a fixed point and on a single axis is known as
    A. circumduction.
    B. opposition.
    C. flexion.
    D. rotation.

14. What word part means below or beneath?
    A. infra-
    B. supra-
    C. hyper-
    D. epi-

15. The word part *cyt-* or *cyte* means what?

    A. cold

    B. small

    C. cell

    D. tissue

16. What word part could be used to identify the innermost layer of tissue in a particular structure?

    A. epi-

    B. peri-

    C. endo-

    D. exo-

17. The liver is an organ located in which quadrant of the abdominopelvic cavity?

    A. upper right

    B. upper left

    C. lower right

    D. lower left

18. The more common term for the cubital region of the body is

    A. shoulder.

    B. arm.

    C. wrist.

    D. elbow.

19. What term refers to *any* disease-causing agent?

    A. pathogen

    B. congenital

    C. virus

    D. bacteria

20. A lung disease caused by inhaling asbestos fibers would be classified as what type of disease?

    A. hereditary

    B. environmental

    C. psychosocial

    D. infectious

21. The specific cause and development of a disease is called the

    A. prognosis.

    B. diagnosis.

    C. etiology.

    D. sequela.

22. A disease with a sudden or rapid onset is said to be a(n) _____ disease.

    A. chronic

    B. congenital

    C. epidemic

    D. acute

23. Tapeworms and lice are examples of which type of pathogen?

    A. parasites

    B. fungi

    C. bacteria

    D. viruses

24. Measles and chicken pox are examples of infections that are also categorized as

    A. autoimmune.

    B. bacterial.

    C. contagious.

    D. nutritional.

25. Multiple sclerosis and rheumatoid arthritis are examples of which category of disease?

    A. noncontagious

    B. autoimmune

    C. environmental

    D. viral

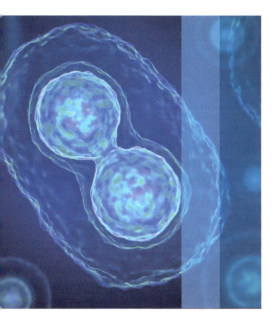

3

Chemistry, Cells, and Tissues

Use this list to choose learning exercises that will help you expand and solidify your understanding of key topics. To test your knowledge, try the Review Quiz at the end of the chapter.

Key Topics	Exercise
• Chemistry Terminology	1
• Basic Cellular Components and Organelles	2–4
• Cellular Transport Mechanisms and Processes	5–6
• Tissues/Histology	7

EXERCISE 1 • Chemistry Crossword

Use this crossword to review and test your ability to define the chemistry terms and concepts from Chapter 3.

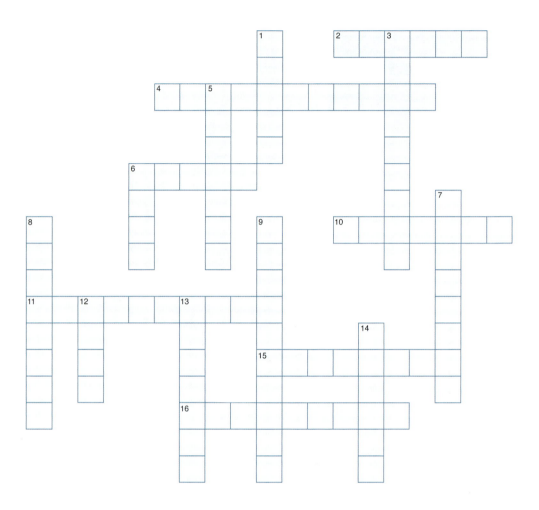

ACROSS

- **2** Fats.
- **4** Another name for an inorganic salt.
- **6** Small invisible units of energy that make up all elements.
- **10** A simple sugar; example of a carbohydrate.
- **11** Proteins are made of chains of these molecules.
- **15** As a free ion, _____ makes substances more acidic.
- **16** Compounds without carbon atoms.

DOWN

- **1** The compound comprised of 2 hydrogen atoms plus 1 oxygen atom.
- **3** Most abundant ion in intracellular fluid.
- **5** A molecule made from identical atoms.
- **6** A substance with a pH below 7.
- **7** A molecule made of two or more different atoms.
- **8** A synonym for basic.
- **9** Nucleic acids differ from proteins because they include these atoms.
- **12** Charged atoms or molecules.
- **13** This ion is important for muscle contraction, blood clotting, and bone structure.
- **14** Na^+.

EXERCISE 2 • Cellular Components Flow Chart

Place the terms into the flow chart to organize the information about cellular components.

centrosome
channel proteins
cytoskeleton
cytosol
DNA
effector proteins
endoplasmic reticulum
genes
genetic blueprint
Golgi apparatus
IMPs
linker proteins
lysosomes
mitochondria
nuclear envelope
nucleolus
organelles
organic compounds
phospholipid
receptor proteins
ribosomes
transport proteins
vesicle

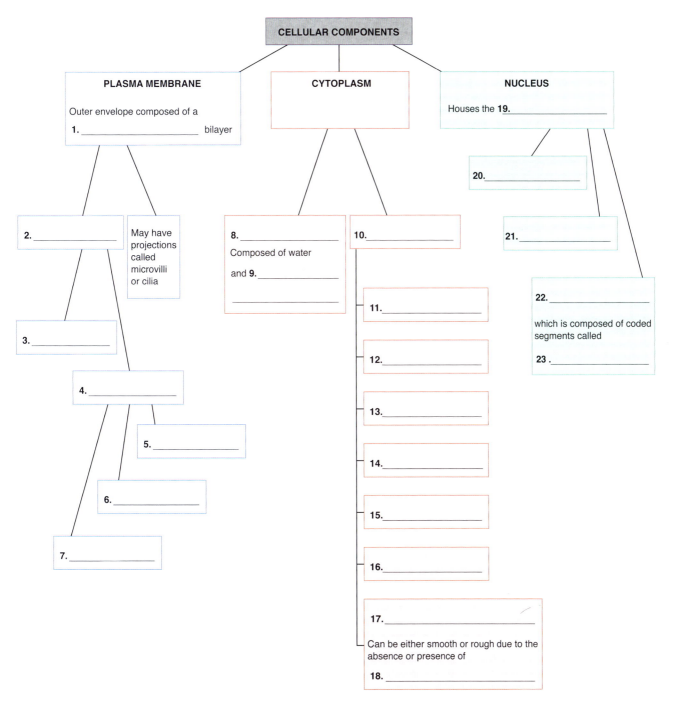

EXERCISE 3 • Cell Diagram

Use this diagram to label the different components of the cell. If you need to refresh your memory, refer to Figure 3.4 in the text.

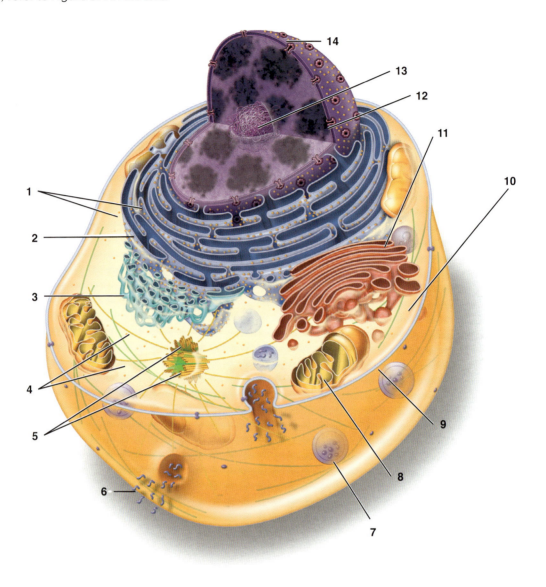

1. _____
2. _____
3. _____
4. _____
5. _____
6. _____
7. _____
8. _____
9. _____
10. _____
11. _____
12. _____
13. _____
14. _____

EXERCISE 4 • A Cell Analogy

Using some of the components listed in Exercises 2 and 3, fill in the blanks to create an analogy for a cell.

A cell is like a city.

- The city limits resemble the **1.** _____ _____ . This boundary
  surrounds the city and controls what comes in and what goes out.

- The town hall is the **2.** _____. It contains the Hall of Records that houses all the
  laws, building blueprints, and other records and is synonymous with the **3.** _____.

- The **4.** _____ are represented by the city's power plants that provide energy
  for the city.

- Because they provide protein, the numerous restaurants found within the city limits are
  5. _____.

- Delivery vehicles are **6.**_____ _____ because they
  package items and deliver them to the city limits to be exported.

- The **7.**_____ of the cell are represented by the dump where food and trash are
  broken down.

- City roads resemble the **8.**_____ _____ because they are
  transportation passageways. Some roads are **9.**_____ with lots of protein factories
  (restaurants, see #5), while others are **10.** _____.

Can you extend the analogy to include other components like IMPs, the centrosome, or the cytoskeleton?

3: Chemistry, Cells, and Tissues   33

EXERCISE 5 • Cellular Transport

Fill in the blanks.

Two-thirds of the total water in the human body can be found inside the cells; this fluid is known as
1. _____ _____. The remaining one-third, called **2.** _____ _____,
makes up the liquid component of blood, lymph, and the fluid that fills the small spaces between cells,
called **3.** _____ _____. This fluid constantly circulates around the cells, providing
a dynamic medium from which nutrients are extracted and wastes released to support cellular activities.
Movement of substances across the cell membrane can be divided into two general categories:

4. _____ Transport—Mechanisms in which the cell does not expend energy because
substances move according to either a concentration or pressure gradient.

5. _____ Transport—Mechanisms that require the cell to use ATP because substances are
being moved against the concentration gradient, engulfed, or secreted.

Which transport mechanisms are represented by the following diagrams?

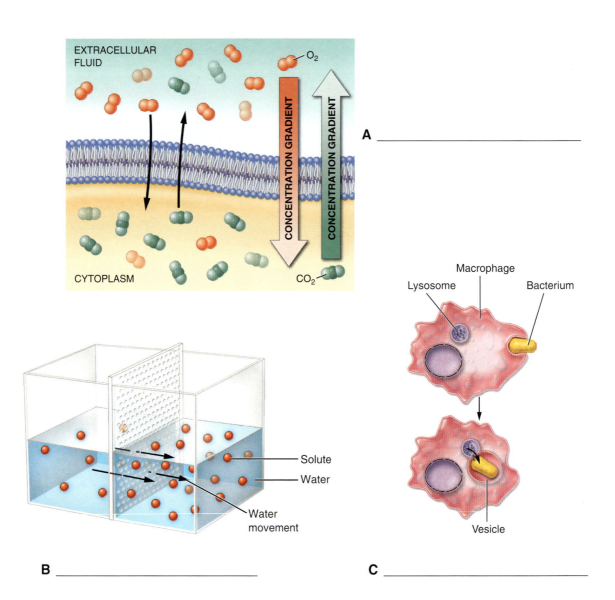

A _____

B _____

C _____

EXERCISE 6 • Cellular Processes Matching

Match the terms with their definitions.

_____ **1.** Metabolism

_____ **2.** Catabolism

_____ **3.** Anabolism

_____ **4.** Protein synthesis

_____ **5.** Glycogen

_____ **6.** Mitosis

_____ **7.** Cytokinesis

_____ **8.** Meiosis

_____ **9.** Differentiation

_____ **10.** Stem cell

_____ **11.** Embryonic layer

_____ **12.** Filtration

_____ **13.** Cell division

_____ **14.** Phagocytosis

_____ **15.** Exocytosis

A. The storage form of glucose

B. The division of cytoplasm

C. A cell that can produce different types of cells

D. Chemical processes

E. Cell eating

F. A process of building up

G. Cellular reproductive process

H. Division of sex cells

I. A process of breaking down or apart

J. Secretion occurs through this process

K. A layer of cells that produces specific tissues

L. Amino acid anabolism

M. Passive transport with the pressure gradient

N. Nuclear division

O. The process of cell specialization

EXERCISE 7 • Histology Concept Map

A concept map is an organizing tool. While similar to a mind map (Chapter 1, Exercises 11 and 12), a concept map goes further by asking you to show the relationship between linked items. Concept maps help you show and explain a hierarchy of information as you describe big ideas with supporting details. Look at the example below. Notice how it shows a flow of information from big ideas to smaller details. Each connecting line or stem is accompanied by a descriptive phrase or linking words that describe the connection represented by the stem.

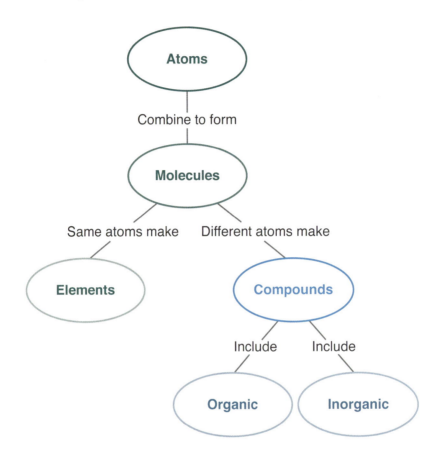

Using the terms and phrases provided, follow the directions to create your own histology concept map that outlines the four types of body tissues. You may want to refer to Tables 3.2 and 3.3 in your text to help with this activity.

Directions:
1. Pick out the largest or main concept(s) from the terms list provided.
2. Categorize the remaining terms and phrases.
3. Within each category, rank the terms and phrases, listing them from general to most specific. Cluster related ideas.
4. Arrange items in a downward flowing or branching structure.
5. Add appropriate linking words or stems (hint: some of the phrases may be used as stems) to describe the connection represented between your terms and phrases.
6. Develop any cross linkages or connecting points you see now that your flow chart has been created.

Terms

adipose	disorganized	liquid	simple
areolar	elastic	loose	skeletal
blood	epithelium	lymph	skeletal muscles
bone	fascia	muscle	skin
brain	fibrocartilage	nerves	smooth (visceral)
cardiac	fibrous	nervous	spinal cord
cartilage	glandular	neurons	spongy
columnar	glial cells	nonconductile	squamous
conductile	heart	nonstriated	stratified
connective	hyaline	organized	striated
cuboidal	involuntary	pseudostratified	tendon
dense	ligament	reticular	voluntary

Phrases

Appearance & nervous system control

Avascular tissue

Cells, fibers & ground substance

Conducts electrical impulses

Covering organs

Lines, covers, protects & secretes

Lining body cavities

Contracts for posture & movement

Shape & arrangement

Supports, connects, protects & transports

Supports, protects & insulates neurons

REVIEW QUIZ

Chemistry, Cells, and Tissues

Multiple Choice: Select the one best answer.

1. The three structural components common to almost all cells are the semipermeable membrane, nucleus, and
   A. cytoplasm.
   B. rough endoplasmic reticulum.
   C. Golgi organs.
   D. centrioles.

2. Which of the following is classified as an inorganic compound?
   A. lipids
   B. nucleic acids
   C. water
   D. carbohydrates

3. A tissue composed of multiple layers of flat epithelial cells would be classified as
   A. pseudostratified.
   B. simple flat.
   C. stratified squamous.
   D. glandular epithelium.

4. Which of the following is an example of loose connective tissue?
   A. tendon
   B. blood
   C. lymph
   D. adipose

5. When two or more like atoms combine to form a molecule, it is called a(n)
   A. compound.
   B. element.
   C. acid.
   D. base.

6. If a compound has a pH below 7, it is
   A. acidic.
   B. alkaline.
   C. neutral.
   D. base.

7. Which organic compound is broken down into amino acids?
   A. carbohydrates
   B. proteins
   C. lipids
   D. starches

8. What is the role of the receptor proteins in the plasma membrane?
   A. shuttle substances across the membrane
   B. monitor the internal and external environment of the cell
   C. regulate the shape and movement of the cell
   D. break down and synthesize various molecules within the cell

9. Which cell organelle is responsible for intracellular transportation?
   A. mitochondria
   B. lysosomes
   C. endoplasmic reticulum
   D. cytoskeleton

10. Which cell organelle is responsible for synthesizing the energy molecule ATP?
    A. lysosomes
    B. ribosomes
    C. mitochondria
    D. endoplasmic reticulum

11. Protein synthesis is the primary function of which organelle?
    A. ribosomes
    B. mitochondria
    C. lysosomes
    D. cytoskeleton

12. What is the term for the passive transport mechanism that moves a substance due to a pressure gradient?
    A. diffusion
    B. filtration
    C. osmosis
    D. phagocytosis

13. What is the name of the diffusion process in which only fluid moves across the semipermeable membrane?
    A. facilitated diffusion
    B. filtration
    C. osmosis
    D. dialysis

14. Which of the following is an example of an active transport mechanism?
    A. facilitated diffusion
    B. osmosis
    C. filtration
    D. sodium pump

15. Which of following is another term for cell division?
    A. differentiation
    B. mitosis
    C. osmosis
    D. splitosis

16. What is the process in which cells begin to specialize into the various types of body cells and tissues?
    A. differentiation
    B. cell division
    C. meiosis
    D. cytolytic mitosis

17. What are the four basic types of tissue in the body?
    A. muscle, skeletal, epithelial, connective
    B. epithelial, muscle, adipose, connective
    C. connective, muscle, adipose, nerve
    D. muscle, epithelial, connective, nerve

18. What are the characteristics that describe visceral muscle tissue?
    A. smooth and involuntary
    B. smooth and voluntary
    C. striated and involuntary
    D. striated and voluntary

19. What type of nerve tissue functions to connect, protect, and support neurons?
    A. neuroglia
    B. neuronal
    C. neuro-connective
    D. neuro-matrix

20. What type of tissue is avascular?
    A. visceral muscle
    B. neuronal
    C. epithelial
    D. loose connective

21. What are the characteristics that describe cardiac muscle tissue?
    A. smooth and involuntary
    B. smooth and voluntary
    C. striated and involuntary
    D. striated and voluntary

22. What is the role of the effector proteins in the plasma membrane of cells?
    A. direct the responses of the cell according to information from receptor proteins
    B. regulate the shape and movement of the cell
    C. monitor the internal environment of the cell to effect changes
    D. provide the cellular identity markers that to help immune system recognize cells as "us"

23. The process of catabolism is defined as
    A. storing of nutrients for future energy needs.
    B. using molecules to repair or build new tissues.
    C. combining cells to form a tissue.
    D. any process used to break down nutrients or molecules.

24. Which type of stem cells are the most limited in their ability to differentiate?
    A. totipotent
    B. pluripotent
    C. multipotent
    D. mesopotent

25. Which type of nerve tissue is conductile?
    A. neuroglia
    B. neuronal
    C. glandular
    D. intercalated

3: Chemistry, Cells, and Tissues

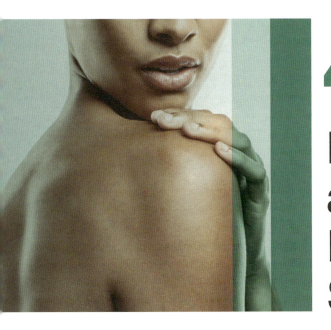

4
Body Membranes and the Integumentary System

Use this list to choose learning exercises that will help you expand and solidify your understanding of key topics. To test your knowledge, try the Review Quiz at the end of the chapter.

Key Topics	Exercise
• System Terminology	1
• Membrane Classification and Characteristics	2 & 3
• Skin Diagram	4
• Integumentary System Components	5–7
• Common Skin Pathologies	8

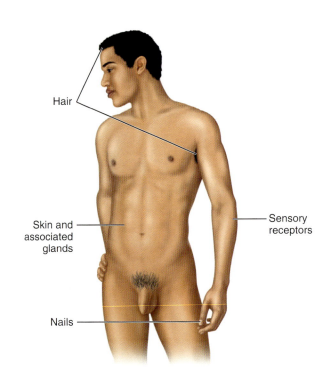

EXERCISE 1 • Terminology Crossword

Use this crossword to review and test your ability to define the terms from Chapter 4.

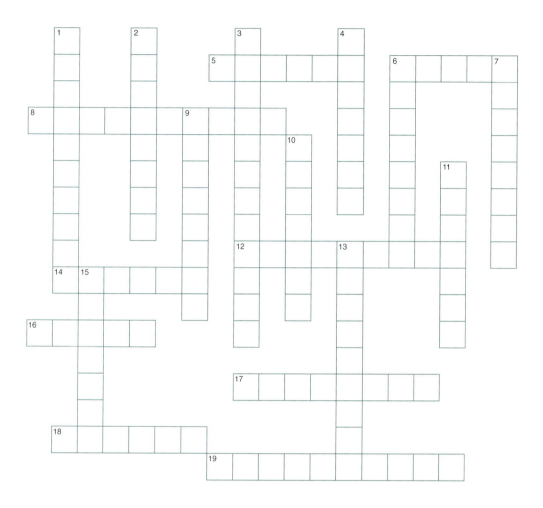

ACROSS

- 5 The arrector pili is a small _____ attached to the hair follicle.
- 6 The oil produced by the sebaceous glands of the skin.
- 8 A free nerve ending sensitive to chemicals released by tissue trauma; a "pain receptor."
- 12 The deeper region of the dermis.
- 14 Layers.
- 16 The thick and clear secretion produced by the membranes that line cavities with openings to the external environment.
- 17 The inner layer of a serous membrane.
- 18 The deeper connective tissue layer of the skin.
- 19 Able to stretch.

DOWN

- 1 The superficial fascia; subcutaneous layer.
- 2 A specialized sweat gland found in the axilla and groin that becomes active at puberty.
- 3 All sweat glands are classified as _____ glands.
- 4 A brown skin pigment.
- 6 A connective tissue membrane that lines joint capsules.
- 7 The most serious type of skin cancer is _____.
- 9 The outer layer of a serous membrane.
- 10 The tough, water-resistant substance found in many cells of the epidermis.
- 11 A common sweat gland.
- 13 This membrane, together with accessory organs, forms the integumentary system.
- 15 This general sense includes the sensations of touch, pressure, vibration, and itch and tickle.

4: Body Membranes and the Integumentary System

EXERCISE 2 • Membranes Organizational Chart

Fill in the blanks of the organizational chart to visually organize the information about body membranes.

MEMBRANES

Definition = 1._____

_____

_____

_____

Broadly classified as

2._____

3._____

includes

includes

4._____	5._____	6._____	7._____
Structure:	**Structure:**	**Structure:**	**Structure:**
Function:	**Function:**	**Function:**	**Function:**
Examples:	**Examples:**	**Examples:**	**Examples:**

EXERCISE 3 • Functional Mnemonic

In Chapter 1, Exercise 4, mnemonics were introduced as helpful memory cues for recalling lists of information. While this is true, learners must be careful to not confuse recall with understanding. Use the list of integumentary system functions in any order to come up with your own mnemonic. Then, explain each function of the skin to be sure you understand what each function entails.

The functions include
- Protection
- Temperature regulation
- Excretion
- Absorption
- General sensory organ
- Synthesis of vitamin D

EXERCISE 4 • Skin Diagram

Label the structures of the integumentary system in this cross section. If you need to refresh your memory, refer to Figure 4.4 in the text.

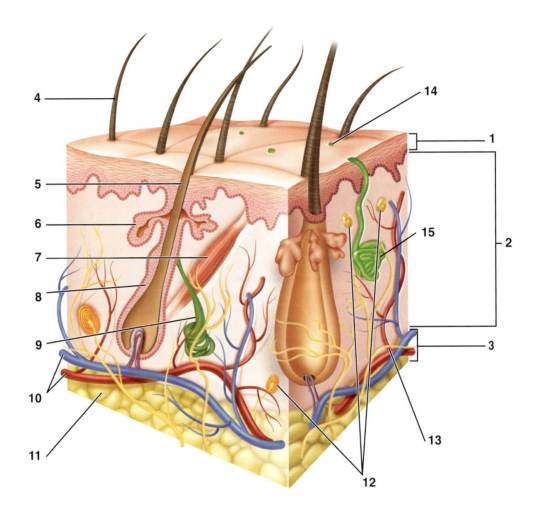

1. _____
2. _____
3. _____
4. _____
5. _____
6. _____
7. _____
8. _____
9. _____
10. _____
11. _____
12. _____
13. _____
14. _____
15. _____

44   REVIEW GUIDE

EXERCISE 5 • Can You Picture It?

Because memories are often stored visually, it can be easier to recall images instead of remembering specific verbal explanations. Instead of structural diagrams and words, try drawing pictures or doodles that represent the functions of each of the following accessory organs of the integumentary system.

Cutaneous receptors

Hair

Nails

Sebaceous gland

Sudoriferous gland

EXERCISE 6 • Matching Structures and Functions

Match the structures below with their specific functions.

_____ **1.** Hair follicle

_____ **2.** Fingernail

_____ **3.** Arrector pili

_____ **4.** Sebaceous gland

_____ **5.** Sudoriferous gland

_____ **6.** Eccrine gland

_____ **7.** Apocrine gland

_____ **8.** Nociceptor

_____ **9.** Merkel disc

_____ **10.** Meissner's corpuscle

_____ **11.** Pacinian corpuscle

_____ **12.** Ruffini's corpuscle

_____ **13.** Hair root plexus

_____ **14.** Sebum

_____ **15.** Epidermis

A. Protects the body from invading pathogens and the sun

B. Sensitive to chemicals released by tissue damage

C. Produces sweat

D. Contracts to raise hairs trapping air for insulation of skin

E. Tube that shapes hair shaft as it grows

F. Sensitive to vibration and light touch

G. Sensitive to deep touch, pressure, and tissue distortion

H. Excretes sweat for thermal and water regulation only

I. Protects fingers; helps us scratch and grasp small objects

J. Senses movement of hair shaft

K. Sensitive to light touch

L. Excretes oil

M. Excretes sweat with traces of lipids and pheromones

N. Sensitive to high-frequency vibrations and deep pressure

O. Lubricates and softens the outer surface of the skin

EXERCISE 7 • Pathology Mind Map

Fill in the mind map to visually organize the information on diseases of the skin. You may want to add items to your map, such as specific examples, signs, or symptoms of some of the skin conditions.

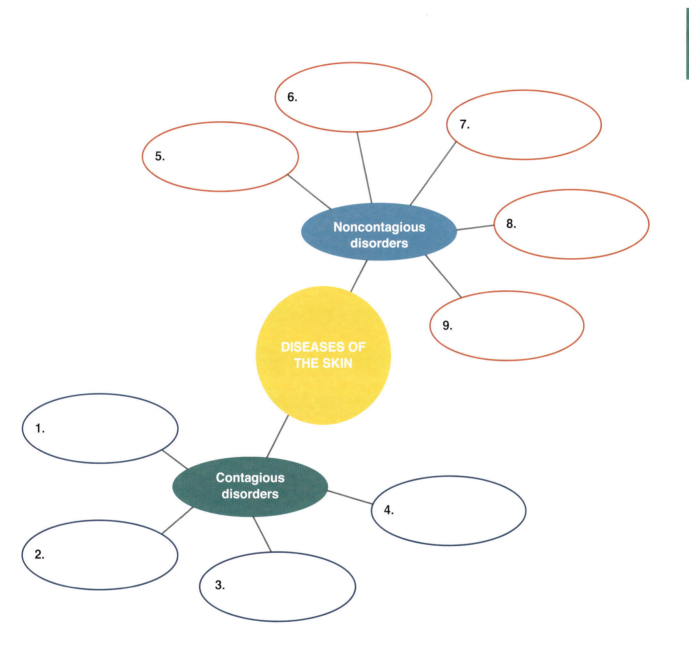

4: Body Membranes and the Integumentary System

EXERCISE 8 • Pestilent Poetry

You may be more comfortable reading and writing poetry and song lyrics than science and medical terminology. Consider applying your talent to help you remember anatomy, physiology, or pathology terms and concepts.

Write a Limerick about Boils or a Sonnet to Psoriasis. Perhaps write a song about the layers of the skin, a cutaneous receptors rap, or rework the functions of the integumentary system as lyrics to the theme song from a favorite TV show or movie. Use your imagination. Here is an example from 18th-century Scottish poet Robert Burns. It's a bit disgusting, but it creates a vivid image.

To a Louse

Ye ugly, creepin, blastit wonner,
Detested, shunn'd by saunt an' sinner,
How daur ye set your fit upon her -
Sae fine a lady!
Gae somewhere else and seek your dinner
On some poor body.

REVIEW QUIZ

Body Membranes and the Integumentary System

Multiple Choice: Select the one best answer.

1. Which of these phrases is the best definition for the term membrane?

  A. a single layer of epithelial tissue that serves as our external covering

  B. two or more layers of tissue that generally serve as coverings or linings to other structures

  C. a group of different cells and tissues working together

  D. four or more layers of tissue that include all four categories of tissue

2. What are the four types of body membranes?

  A. connective, nervous, epithelial, muscular

  B. serous, connective, epithelial, areolar

  C. synovial, mucous, cutaneous, serous

  D. cutaneous, synovial, connective, areolar

3. The primary functions of the integumentary system are to serve as a protective covering, help regulate body temperature, _____, and _____.

  A. produce vitamin K; maintain water balance

  B. produce essential oils for flexibility; secrete metabolic wastes

  C. serve as large sensory organ; produce vitamin D

  D. serve as largest storage site for energy; regulate water usage

4. What is the name for the serous membrane covering the outside of the lungs?

  A. parietal peritoneum

  B. visceral peritoneum

  C. parietal pleura

  D. visceral pleura

5. The general sensory receptors found in the skin include nociceptors, Meissner's corpuscles, hair root plexuses, Pacinian corpuscles, _____ , and_____.

  A. free nerve endings; Merkle discs

  B. cutaneous corpuscles; pain receptors

  C. thermoreceptors; olfactory sensors

  D. Merrill discs; synovial plexuses

6. The _____ membrane, plus its associated accessory organs, makes up the integumentary system.

  A. synovial

  B. serous

  C. cutaneous

  D. mucous

7. What is the name of the most superficial layer of skin?

  A. dermis

  B. epidermis

  C. integument

  D. superficial fascia

8. The deepest layer of the epidermis is called the _____ layer because that is where the epithelial cells are produced.

  A. germinating

  B. horny

  C. granular

  D. spiny

9. What is the function of keratin?

  A. lubricate and soften the skin

  B. eliminate heat and metabolic byproducts

  C. toughen and waterproof the skin

  D. protect the skin from UV radiation

10. Which substance in skin determines its color?

  A. keratin

  B. sebum

  C. corneum

  D. melanin

11. Which of the following is a defining characteristic of the epidermis?

  A. contains many accessory organs

  B. composed of numerous layers of epithelial cells

  C. has a rich blood supply

  D. provides energy storage

12. Which layer of skin is primarily connective tissue and contains nerves and blood and lymph vessels?

  A. epidermis

  B. dermis

  C. hypodermis

  D. superficial fascia

13. What is the name of the most superficial layer/region of the dermis?
    A. hyperdermis
    B. stratum corneum
    C. exodermis
    D. papillary

14. What is the role and function of the hypodermis?
    A. insulation and energy storage
    B. protection and sebum production
    C. secretion of metabolic byproducts
    D. synthesis of vitamin D

15. Which of the following glands produce oil to keep skin soft?
    A. sudoriferous
    B. sebaceous
    C. apocrine
    D. eccrine

16. What types of glands are found only in certain areas of the body such as the axilla and groin?
    A. sebaceous
    B. eccrine
    C. apocrine
    D. nociceptors

17. What is the most numerous and widespread cutaneous receptor?
    A. Merkel discs
    B. Pacinian corpuscles
    C. hair root plexuses
    D. free nerve endings

18. Which of the accessory organs is most responsible for creating the temperature and water regulation function of our skin?
    A. apocrine glands
    B. Pacinian corpuscles
    C. eccrine glands
    D. sebaceous glands

19. Which of these specific sensations is properly categorized as a touch or tactile sense?
    A. hot
    B. acute pain
    C. vibration
    D. olfaction

20. What is the term for an area of skin that is innervated by the branches of a specific spinal nerve?
    A. dermatome
    B. myotome
    C. enterotome
    D. neuraltome

21. Two noncontagious skin conditions are eczema and
    A. tinea cruris.
    B. ringworm.
    C. impetigo.
    D. vitiligo.

22. What is the proper medical term for athlete's foot?
    A. herpes pedis
    B. vitiligo
    C. tinea pedis
    D. urticaria

23. Herpes zoster is more commonly known as
    A. shingles.
    B. ringworm.
    C. boils.
    D. mouth sores.

24. What are the two most common parasitic skin conditions?
    A. eczema and psoriasis
    B. scabies and lice
    C. hives and acne
    D. MRSA and carbuncles

25. Which of these bacterial infections is antibiotic resistant?
    A. herpes simplex 2
    B. MRSA
    C. tinea corporis
    D. cellulitis

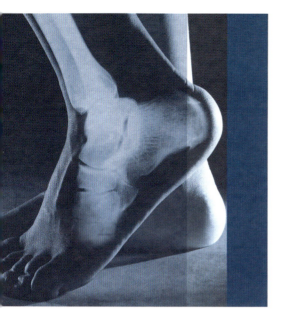

5

The Skeletal System

Use this list to choose learning exercises that will help you expand and solidify your understanding of key topics. To test your knowledge, try the Review Quiz at the end of the chapter.

Key Topics	Exercise
• System Terminology	1
• Functions of the System	2
• The Skeleton	3
• Bones and Their Parts	4–6
• Bone Landmarks	7
• Synovial Joints: Types, Structures, and Movements	8–10

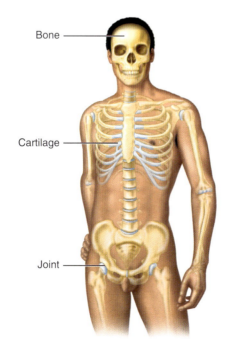

EXERCISE 1 • Bony Terms Crossword

Use this crossword to review and test your ability to define the bone and landmark terms from Chapter 5.

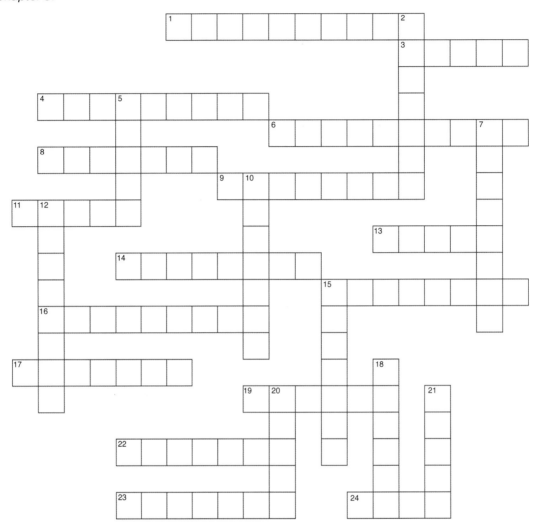

ACROSS

1. The heel bone.
3. Shin bone.
4. The point of the elbow; proximal posterior ulna.
6. A large bump such as the one on the tibia where the quadriceps attach.
8. Upper arm bone.
9. The butterfly-shaped internal cranial bone.
11. A small flat articulating surface.
13. Thigh bone.
14. The collar bone.
15. Jaw bone.
16. A projection at the distal tibia or the fibula; "ankle bones."
17. A rounded projection at the end of the bone, often a point of articulation.
19. The fused ilium, ischium, and pubic bones; one side of the pelvis.
22. A hole in a bone for blood vessels or nerves.
23. The posterior process of a spinal vertebra.
24. Medial forearm bone.

DOWN

2. A needle-like process.
5. A sharp ridge.
7. A small bump such as the one on the humerus where the deltoid attaches.
10. A prominent projection.
12. Point of the shoulder; lateral projection of the scapula.
15. A process on the temporal bone just posterior to the ear.
18. A wrist bone.
20. A bone cavity.
21. A large saucer-shaped depression.

EXERCISE 2 • A Story of Functions

When you want to recall something specific, it is helpful to have a context for remembering. For example, when many of us want to remember the alphabet, we sing "The Alphabet Song," or when we want to recall the face of a loved one, we picture them doing something specific like laughing at a joke, playing ball, or doing the dishes. As learners, we can create context for important information by inserting facts into a story, drawing, poem, or song.

Try writing a story or play where the characters are responsible for the functions of the skeletal system, or use the same information to write a poem or lyrics for a song.

EXERCISE 3 • Label the Skeleton

Using two different colors, identify the axial and appendicular portions of the skeleton on the diagrams. Then label each of the numbered bones. If you need to refresh your memory, refer to Figure 5.1 in your text. Write the name of each bone in the space provided.

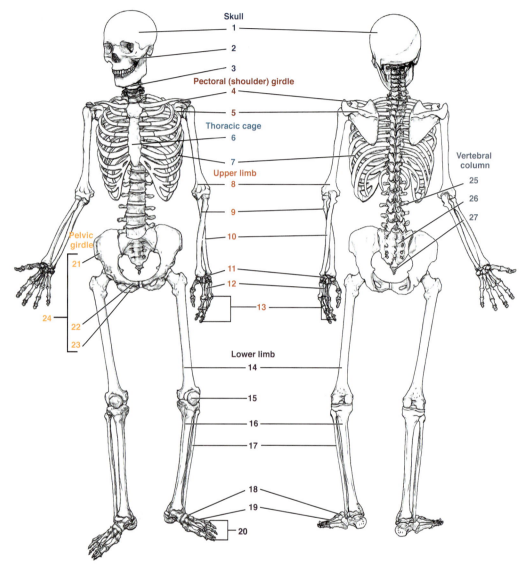

1. _____
2. _____
3. _____
4. _____
5. _____
6. _____
7. _____
8. _____
9. _____
10. _____
11. _____
12. _____
13. _____
14. _____
15. _____
16. _____
17. _____
18. _____
19. _____
20. _____
21. _____
22. _____
23. _____
24. _____
25. _____
26. _____
27. _____

EXERCISE 4 • Draw Me a Bone

Using the table below, list the four bone shapes in the column headed SHAPE. Then, in the spaces provided, draw a picture of each bone shape and list at least one example of each. Refer to Figure 5.3 in the textbook if you need to refresh your memory.

SHAPE	PICTURE	EXAMPLES

5: The Skeletal System

EXERCISE 5 • Parts of a Long Bone

Match the parts of a long bone with their description and/or function. Next, label the diagram of the long bone below. If you need to refresh your memory, refer to Figure 5.4 in your textbook.

_____ 1. Epiphysis
_____ 2. Articular cartilage
_____ 3. Red bone marrow
_____ 4. Epiphyseal line
_____ 5. Spongy bone
_____ 6. Metaphysis
_____ 7. Diaphysis
_____ 8. Periosteum
_____ 9. Endosteum
_____ 10. Medullary cavity
_____ 11. Yellow bone marrow
_____ 12. Compact bone

A. Site of bone elongation; growth plate
B. Tough outer connective tissue covering
C. Bone end
D. Fatty tissue in medullary cavity
E. Region between epiphysis and diaphysis
F. Hematopoietic tissue
G. Comprises the shaft
H. Space in the middle of the shaft
I. Covers and protects bone ends; hyaline
J. Shaft of the long bone
K. Comprises the bone ends
L. Inner lining of the medullary cavity

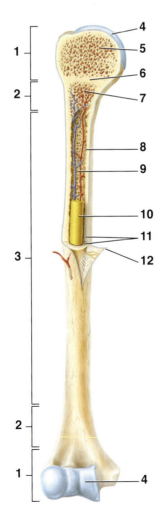

1. _____
2. _____
3. _____
4. _____
5. _____
6. _____
7. _____
8. _____
9. _____
10. _____
11. _____
12. _____

56   REVIEW GUIDE

EXERCISE 6 • Build a Long Bone

Another way to learn about the structure of something is to make a model using simple materials you can get at any home improvement store. For example, to build a model of a long bone, you can use the following:

- A 6- to 12-inch length of 1-inch PVC piping
- Two caps to fit on the ends of your PVC pipe
- Silly Putty
- Elastic food wrap
- Pink/red sponge pieces
- Yellow sponge pieces

Once you have gathered all your materials, construct your model. Fill in the blanks below to identify which materials represent the individual parts of a long bone.

The length of pipe represents the **1.**_____, or shaft of the bone. Therefore, the space

inside is the **2.**_____ _____ that contains **3.**_____

_____ _____. This tissue is represented by the yellow sponge pieces that

you can place inside the pipe. The PVC caps represent the ends of the bone, or **4.**_____,

where the **5.**_____ _____ _____ resides. Stuff the caps

with pink/red sponge pieces and attach them to the shaft. Use some Silly Putty to cover the very ends of the

model to represent the **6.**_____ _____ that protects the bone ends from

wear and tear during movement. Then wrap the entire length of the bone with elastic wrap to represent the

7._____, the connective tissue sheath that surrounds the bone.

5: The Skeletal System   57

EXERCISE 7 • Skeletal Landmarks Labeling

Match the bone or landmark with its label on the diagram.

_____ 1. Iliac crest

_____ 2. Lateral malleolus

_____ 3. Greater trochanter

_____ 4. Occipital bone

_____ 5. Olecranon process

_____ 6. Calcaneus

_____ 7. Patella

_____ 8. Inferior angle of scapula

_____ 9. Mastoid process

_____ 10. Acromion process

_____ 11. Mandible

_____ 12. Tibial tuberosity

_____ 13. Head of radius

_____ 14. Anterior superior iliac spine

_____ 15. Ischial tuberosity

_____ 16. Glenoid fossa

_____ 17. Spinous process

_____ 18. Lateral humeral epicondyle

_____ 19. Xiphoid process

_____ 20. Crest of tibia

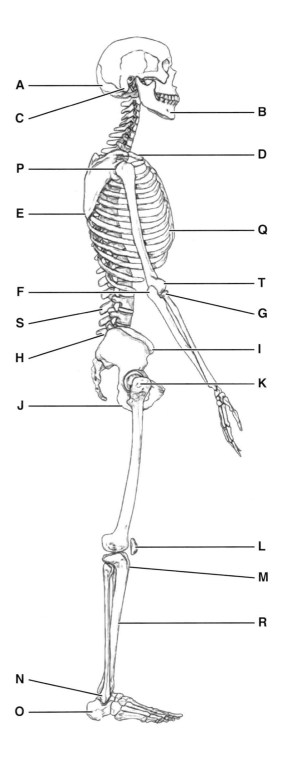

EXERCISE 8 • Label a Synovial Joint

All synovial or diarthrotic joints share some common structural components. Label the sagittal section of the knee provided to review the structures of a synovial joint. If you need to refresh your memory, refer to Figure 5.24 in your textbook.

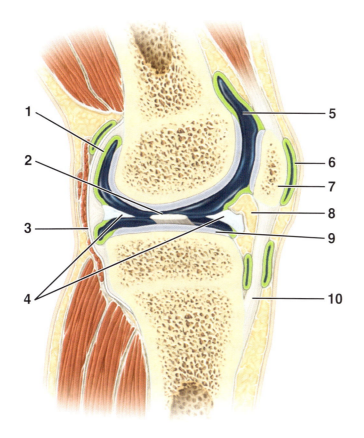

1. _____
2. _____
3. _____
4. _____
5. _____
6. _____
7. _____
8. _____
9. _____
10. _____

Anterior cruciate ligament
Articular cartilage
Bursa
Fat pad
Fibrous joint capsule
Menisci
Patella
Patellar ligament
Synovial fluid
Synovial membrane

EXERCISE 9 • Diarthrotic Joint Movements

Complete the table below by identifying the type of joint and the movements allowed by each specific joint listed. The first one is done for you.

SPECIFIC JOINT	TYPE	MOVEMENTS
Atlantooccipital joint	Hinge	Flexion/extension
Atlantoaxial	1.	2.
Glenohumeral	3.	4.
Radioulnar	5.	6.
Humeroulnar	7.	8.
Radiocarpal	9.	10.
First carpometacarpal	11.	12.
Metacarpophalangeal	13.	14.
Interphalangeal	15.	16.
Iliofemoral	17.	18.
Femorotibial (knee)	19.	20.
Tibiotalar (ankle)	21.	22.
Talotarsal (subtalar)	23.	24.

60   REVIEW GUIDE

EXERCISE 10 • Joint Crossword

Use this crossword to review and test your knowledge about joint classifications, names, and movements.

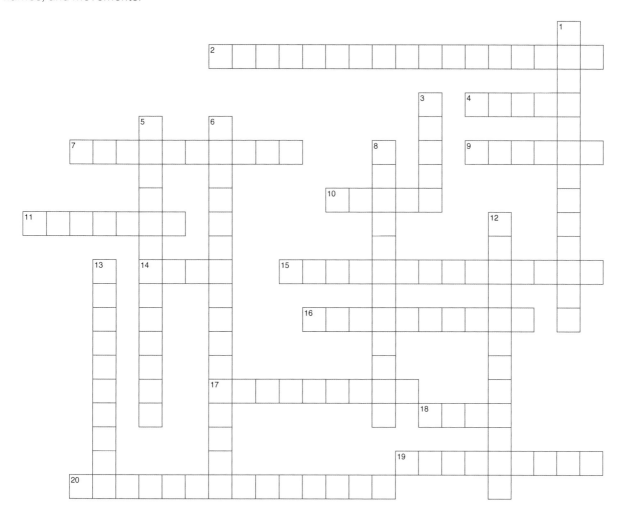

ACROSS

2. The TM in TMJ.
4. A synovial joint that allows rotation only.
7. Turning the forearm so that the palm faces forward in anatomic position.
9. The joint category that includes the first carpometacarpal joint.
10. A diarthosis that allows flexion and extension only.
11. The structural joint category that includes the sutures of the skull.
14. A fibrocartilage pad found between vertebrae; intervertebral ____.
15. Rising up on the toes.
16. To draw a body part backward.
17. A synovial joint that allows movement in the frontal and sagittal planes.
18. The tibiofemoral joint.
19. Upward movement.
20. Slightly movable joint.

DOWN

1. The structural joint category that includes the pubic symphysis.
3. The tibiotalar joint.
5. Multiplanar movement where the distal end of a limb makes a circle and the proximal end serves as a single fixed point.
6. The joint between the manubrium and clavicle.
8. Immovable joint.
12. The shoulder joint.
13. The hip socket.

5: The Skeletal System

REVIEW QUIZ

The Skeletal System

Multiple Choice: Select the one best answer.

1. The five functions of the skeletal system are providing framework for the body and levers for movement, producing blood cells, _____, and _____.
   A. storing vitamin D; producing calcium
   B. creating movement; storing vitamin C
   C. protecting vital organs; storing calcium and minerals
   D. providing the fulcrums for movement; storing energy

2. The five types of bones are long, short, sesamoid, _____, and _____.
   A. irregular; cylindrical
   B. square; cuboid
   C. cylindrical; flat
   D. flat; irregular

3. What is the structural classification for joints that are partially moveable?
   A. cartilaginous
   B. synovial
   C. fibrous
   D. synarthrotic

4. Which of the six different types of synovial joints allows all five of the basic movements?
   A. hinge
   B. condyloid
   C. pivot
   D. ball-and-socket

5. Which of the six different types of synovial joints allows flexion and extension only?
   A. condyloid
   B. hinge
   C. gliding
   D. ellipsoid

6. Which category of joint is described as immoveable?
   A. ellipsoid
   B. synarthrosis
   C. gliding
   D. synovial

7. Which of these is classified as an axial bone?
   A. radius
   B. clavicle
   C. sacrum
   D. scapula

8. Which of these is considered an appendicular bone?
   A. scapula
   B. sternum
   C. skull
   D. rib

9. Which of these is a facial bone?
   A. parietal
   B. lacrimal
   C. sphenoid
   D. sesamoid

10. What is the anatomic term for the collar bone?
    A. costal
    B. zygomatic
    C. clavicle
    D. scapula

11. What is the anatomic name for the bones of our fingers and toes?
    A. metacarpals
    B. phalanges
    C. fontanels
    D. tarsals

12. What are the anatomic names for the ends of long bones?
    A. epiphyses
    B. diaphysis
    C. epiphyseal plate
    D. medullary ends

13. What type of bone tissue gives the shaft of a long bone its strength?
    A. compact
    B. spongy
    C. trabeculae
    D. cancellous

62 REVIEW GUIDE

14. The hollow cavity in the shaft of a long bone is called the _____ cavity.
    A. diaphysis
    B. yellow marrow
    C. epiphyseal
    D. medullary

15. Blood cell production occurs in what part of the bone?
    A. medullary cavity
    B. epiphysis
    C. diaphysis
    D. periosteum

16. What type of tissue covers the articular surface of the bone ends?
    A. fibrocartilage
    B. hyaline cartilage
    C. periosteum
    D. synovial membrane

17. What bone in the lower extremity is considered to be non–weight-bearing?
    A. femur
    B. tibia
    C. fibula
    D. talus

18. How many vertebrae make up the cervical region of the spinal column?
    A. 10
    B. 5
    C. 7
    D. 9

19. How many pairs of "true ribs" do we have in our rib cage?
    A. 7
    B. 10
    C. 12
    D. 5

20. What is the term for the most proximal portion of the sternum that articulates with the clavicle?
    A. body
    B. xyphoid process
    C. coracoid process
    D. manubrium

21. Which of the following joints is amphiarthrotic?
    A. acromioclavicular
    B. atlantoaxial
    C. pubic symphysis
    D. intervertebral facet joints

22. Which of the following is the best example of a condyloid joint?
    A. metacarpophalangeal
    B. proximal radioulnar
    C. distal interphalangeal
    D. iliofemoral

23. What is the name of the flat shelf-like process projecting from the lateral end of the spine of the scapula?
    A. coracoid
    B. coranoid
    C. acromion
    D. deltoid

24. What is another term for dense or compact bone tissue?
    A. cancellous
    B. trabeculae
    C. lacunae
    D. cortical

25. The group of concentric rings that make up compact bone is called an osteon, or _____ system.
    A. haversian
    B. trabecular
    C. osseous
    D. cancellous

5: The Skeletal System   63

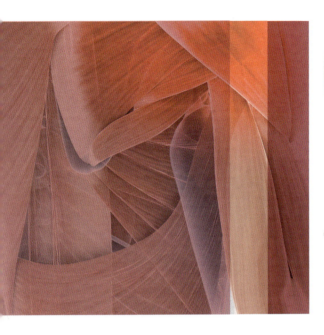

6

The Skeletal Muscle System

Use this list to choose learning exercises that will help you expand and solidify your understanding of key topics. To test your knowledge, try the Review Quiz at the end of the chapter.

Key Topics	Exercise
• System Terminology	1
• Major Parts of a Skeletal Muscle	2
• Fascia and Tendons	3
• Skeletal Muscle Fiber Organization	4 & 5
• Skeletal Muscle Contraction	6
• Energy for Contraction	7 & 8
• Architecture of Skeletal Muscles	9
• Muscle Movement Assignments	10 & 14
• Naming and Locating Muscles	11 – 14

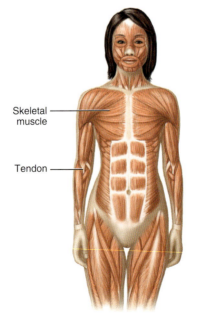

64

EXERCISE 1 • Muscle Terminology Crossword

Use this crossword to review and test your knowledge of the general muscle anatomy and physiology terms from Chapter 6.

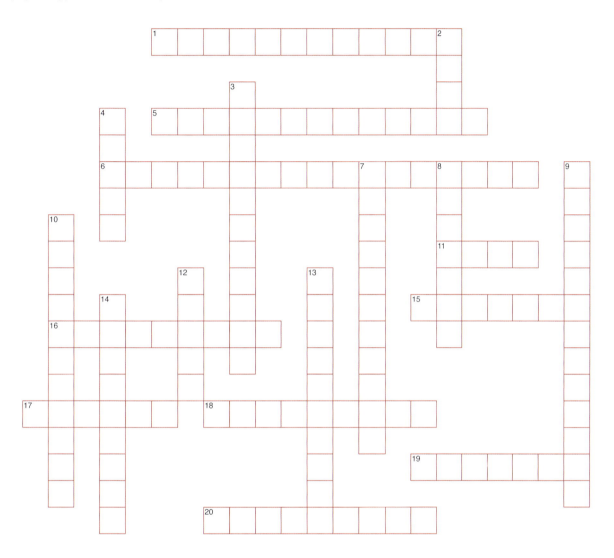

ACROSS

1. Type of fibrous connective tissue that makes up fascia.
5. The region of a muscle fiber that is highly sensitive to neurotransmitters.
6. Communicating chemicals released from a neuron.
11. The breakdown of ATP in muscle produces this byproduct, which is why we shiver when we are cold.
15. Able to rebound back to original shape and length.
16. Highly responsive to stimulation from the nervous system.
17. Muscles work together with ligaments and joint capsules to stabilize _____.
18. The minimum stimulus required to produce a response.
19. Inability to contract forcefully after prolonged activity.
20. A muscle contraction in which there is an increase in tension, but no change in length.

DOWN

2. The oxygen required by the body to metabolize lactic acid and replenish glycogen, creatine phosphate, and ATP stores after exercise.
3. Capable of forcefully shortening.
4. The type of contraction responsible for maintaining posture.
7. A nerve cell that stimulates multiple muscle fibers in a motor unit.
8. The organized fibrous connective tissue that makes up tendons is composed of _____ packed collagen fibers.
9. Corkscrew-shaped protein that composes collagen fibrils.
10. A broad, flat sheet of organized connective tissue that attaches a muscle to bone.
12. An acute involuntary muscle contraction that lasts for several minutes; palpable as a knot.
13. Able to lengthen.
14. An isotonic contraction in which the muscle produces tension while it is lengthening.

6: The Skeletal Muscle System

EXERCISE 2 • Major Parts of a Skeletal Muscle

Color and label the diagram to identify the major parts of a skeletal muscle. Consider using different colors to distinguish the different layers of fascia within the muscle. Refer to Figure 6.1 in the textbook if you need to refresh your memory.

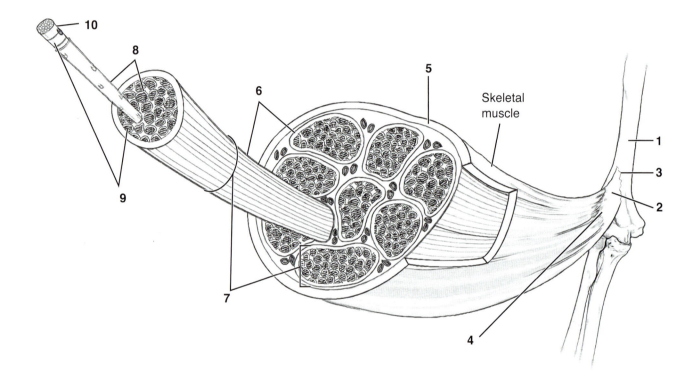

1. _____
2. _____
3. _____
4. _____
5. _____
6. _____
7. _____
8. _____
9. _____
10. _____

EXERCISE 3 • Comparing Fascia and Tendons

Venn diagrams are simple graphic organizers that provide a visual display of similar and different attributes between two items or sets of information. Each circle in the diagram represents one item or set of information. Where the circles overlap, characteristics that are shared between the two items are recorded. Characteristics that differ between the items are recorded in the areas where the circles do not overlap.

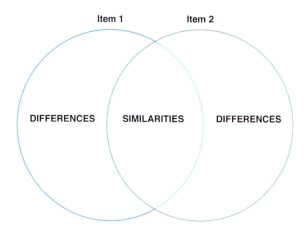

Use the Venn diagram below to compare and contrast the structural and functional characteristics of fascia and tendons. An example of one shared characteristic—that is, composed of fibrous connective tissue—has been placed in the area of overlap to get you started.

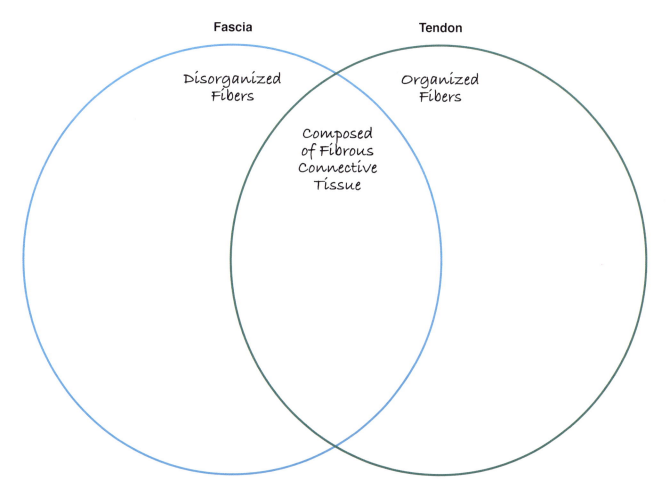

6: The Skeletal Muscle System   67

EXERCISE 4 • Skeletal Muscle Fiber Organization

Match each organizational component with its definition or functional description. Refer to Figure 6.2 in the textbook if you need to refresh your memory.

_____ **1.** Muscle fiber

_____ **2.** Myofibrils

_____ **3.** Mitochondrion

_____ **4.** Sarcoplasmic reticulum

_____ **5.** Sarcolemma

_____ **6.** Myofilaments

_____ **7.** Myosin

_____ **8.** Actin

_____ **9.** Z line

_____ **10.** A band

_____ **11.** I band

_____ **12.** Sarcomere

A. The ER of a muscle fiber

B. The thin myofilament

C. Light area of sarcomere; contains thin filaments only

D. Small cylindrical organelles that make up a fiber

E. Actin and myosin

F. A muscle cell

G. The functional unit of contraction

H. Dark area of a sarcomere created by thick filaments

I. The thick myofilament

J. Many found in each muscle cell to produce ATP

K. The plasma membrane of a muscle fiber

L. Boundary between two sarcomeres

68   REVIEW GUIDE

EXERCISE 5 • Muscle Microanatomy

Use the key terms from Exercise 4 to label the microanatomy diagram below.

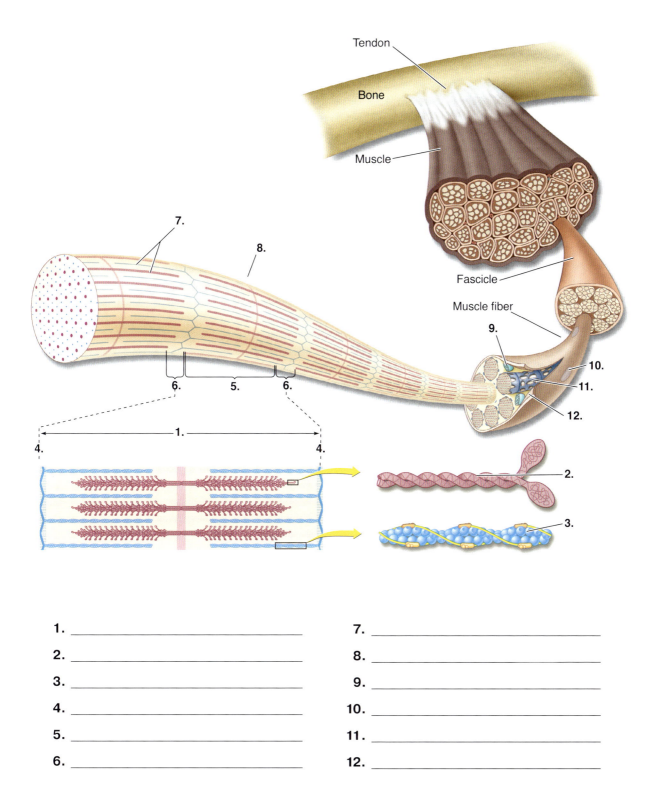

1. _____
2. _____
3. _____
4. _____
5. _____
6. _____
7. _____
8. _____
9. _____
10. _____
11. _____
12. _____

EXERCISE 6 • Skeletal Muscle Contraction

Fill in the blanks to describe the process of muscle contraction.

The physiology of muscle contraction is explained through a model called the **1.**_____ _____

_____. This model lays out the key physiologic events that create the shortening of the

2._____when muscle cells are signaled to contract by the nervous system. The

coordination between the nervous and muscular systems occurs through the functional structure called a

3._____, which is composed of a **4.**_____ and the

multiple muscle **5.**_____ it innervates. The structural interface between these

structures is a microscopic space called the **6.**_____. A muscle contraction

is initiated when **7.**_____ are released from the vesicles in the knobs of the

8._____ into this space or junction to stimulate the **9.**_____

_____ of the muscle fibers.

A contraction only occurs when enough stimulation is delivered to the fibers. This minimum amount of

stimulus is called a **10.**_____. A physiological principle known as **11.** _____

_____ applies to each individual motor unit. This principle states that if **12.** _____

is reached, **13.** _____ the muscle fibers in the motor unit will fully contract. If not, **14.** _____

of the fibers will contract. The nervous system regulates the force of muscle contraction by controlling the

number of motor units stimulated within any given muscle. The regulation of a muscle's effort by increasing or

decreasing the number of motor units stimulated is called **15.**_____, or

16._____.

When a muscle is stimulated, the steps of muscle contraction are as follows:

- **17.**_____ ions stored in the **18.**_____ are released
  into the sarcoplasm.

- The presence of these ions exposes binding sites on the **19.**_____

- The **20.**_____ bind to these exposed sites, forming cross bridges that
  21. _____

- ATP is used to detach the **22.**_____ so that they can flip forward to the next
  binding site. The net result is **23.** _____

- When the stimulus is removed, more energy is expended to pump **24.**_____
  back into the **25.**_____ and chemical bridges can no longer form.

70   REVIEW GUIDE

EXERCISE 7 • Picturing Energy for Muscle Contraction

Label the diagrams to review the three methods of energy production for muscle contraction.
If you need to refresh your memory, refer to Figures 6.7 and 6.8 in the text.

Direct Phosphorylation

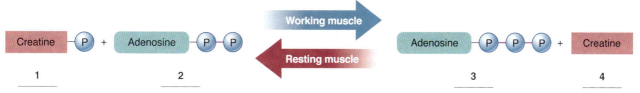

Glycolysis and Aerobic Cellular Metabolism

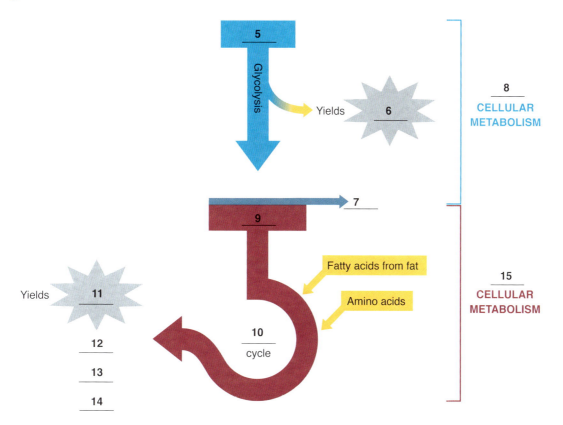

1. _____
2. _____
3. _____
4. _____
5. _____
6. _____
7. _____
8. _____
9. _____
10. _____
11. _____
12. _____
13. _____
14. _____
15. _____

EXERCISE 8 • Organizing Methods of ATP Production

Use the table below to organize the key information about the three methods of ATP production for muscle contraction.

Energy for Muscle Contraction

METHOD	DESCRIPTION	O_2 NEEDED?	BYPRODUCTS
1.	Phosphate from creatine phosphate attaches to ADP to create ATP for short burst of activity.	No, anaerobic process	2.
GLYCOLYSIS	3.	4.	ATP and pyruvic acid. Without oxygen, pyruvic acid converts to lactic acid.
5.	6.	Yes, aerobic process	7.

EXERCISE 9 • Types of Fiber Arrangements

Muscles have a variety of fascicle or fiber arrangements that are an important part of their overall architecture. Complete the table on types of fiber arrangements by drawing a picture and providing at least one example of each. Refer to Figure 6.11 in the text if you need to refresh your memory.

Fiber Arrangements

	ARRANGEMENT	PICTURE	EXAMPLE(S)
PARALLEL	Parallel		1.
	2.		Biceps brachii Biceps femoris
	3.		Orbicularis oris Orbicularis oculi
	Triangular		4.
PENNATE	Unipennate		5.
	6.		Rectus femoris External obliques
	7.		Deltoid Triceps brachii

72   REVIEW GUIDE

EXERCISE 10 • Muscle Assignments

Define the following muscle assignments:

Agonist (prime mover)_____

_____

Antagonist _____

_____

Synergist _____

_____

Stabilizer _____

_____

Next, complete the table by providing at least one agonist, antagonist, and synergist for each movement.

MOVEMENT		PRIME MOVER	ANTAGONIST	SYNERGIST
KNEE	Extension	Rectus femoris	**1.**	**2.**
	Flexion	**3.**	**4.**	Semimembranosus Semitendinosus Gastrocnemius
SHOULDER	Extension	**5.**	Pectoralis major Coracobrachialis	Teres major
	Flexion	**6.**	**7.**	**8.**
	Abduction	**9.**	**10.**	Supraspinatus
	Adduction	Pectoralis major	**11.**	**12.**
	Medial rotation	Subscapularis	**13.**	Pectoralis major Latissimus dorsi
	Lateral rotation	Infraspinatus	**14.**	**15.**

6: The Skeletal Muscle System

EXERCISE 11 • Naming Muscles

Use the mind map to show typical themes among muscle names. Provide as many examples as you can for each. An example has been provided to get you started.

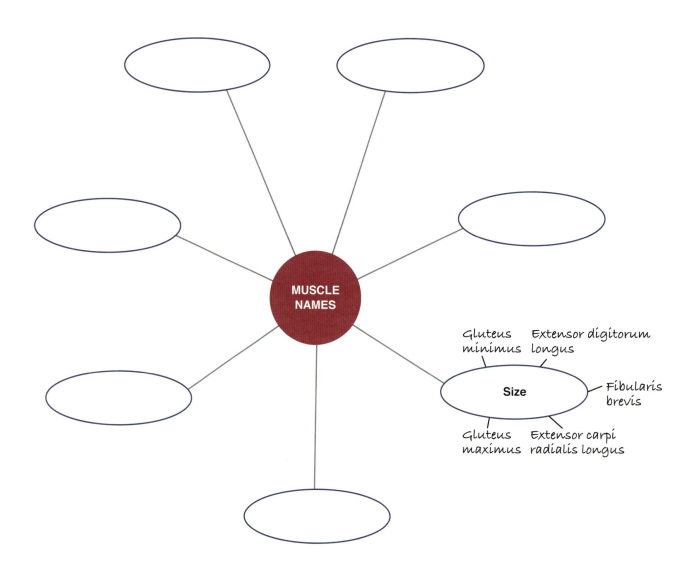

EXERCISE 12 • Locating Major Muscles

Complete the diagrams by coloring and labeling the major muscles. Consider using a variety of colors to help you easily differentiate neighboring muscles. If you wish to refresh your memory, refer to Figures 6.12 and 6.13 in the textbook.

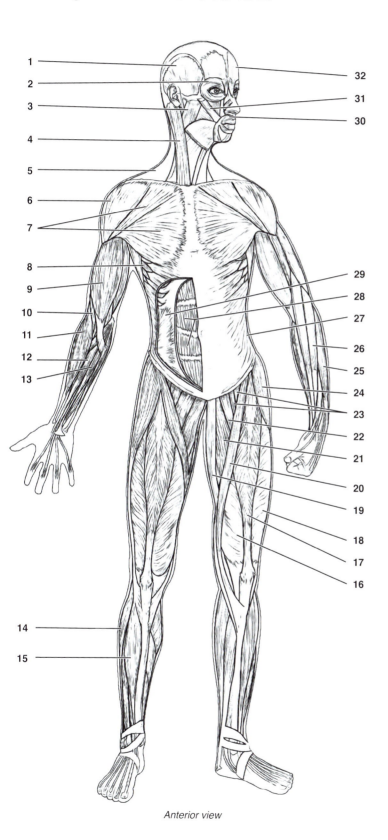

Anterior view

1. _____
2. _____
3. _____
4. _____
5. _____
6. _____
7. _____
8. _____
9. _____
10. _____
11. _____
12. _____
13. _____
14. _____
15. _____
16. _____
17. _____
18. _____
19. _____
20. _____
21. _____
22. _____
23. _____
24. _____
25. _____
26. _____
27. _____
28. _____
29. _____
30. _____
31. _____
32. _____

6: The Skeletal Muscle System 75

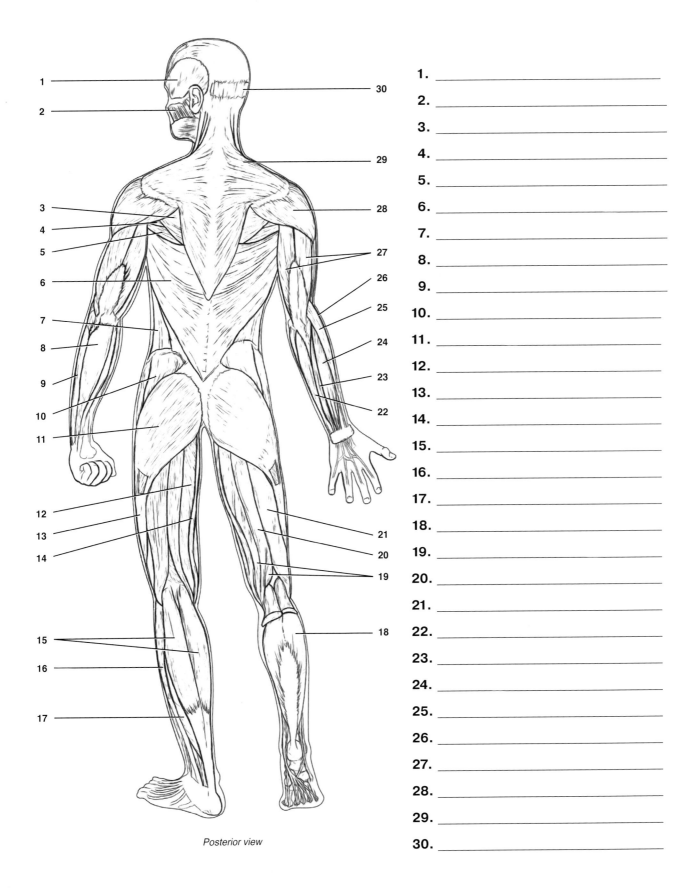

Posterior view

1. _____
2. _____
3. _____
4. _____
5. _____
6. _____
7. _____
8. _____
9. _____
10. _____
11. _____
12. _____
13. _____
14. _____
15. _____
16. _____
17. _____
18. _____
19. _____
20. _____
21. _____
22. _____
23. _____
24. _____
25. _____
26. _____
27. _____
28. _____
29. _____
30. _____

76 REVIEW GUIDE

EXERCISE 13 • Building Muscles

It can help to use a model to learn origins and insertions and understand the actions of muscles. By molding clay or placing scarves, fabric cutouts, or therapeutic exercise bands on a skeleton, you can identify a muscle's specific location and see how it crosses joints to produce movement.

Use the recipe below to make large amounts of homemade play dough. Using a skeleton of any size, mold muscles from play dough onto the skeleton. Consider making several batches in different colors to layer muscles in the same region of the body. For example, to see how the three primary elbow flexors overlap one another in the elbow, make the brachialis one color, the biceps brachii another, and the brachioradialis a third.

Homemade Play Dough

- Mix 2½ cups flour, ½ cup salt, and 1 tablespoon alum thoroughly.
- Make a well in the middle of these dry ingredients and pour 3 tablespoons corn oil, 2 cups boiling water, and food coloring into the well.
- Stir well and then knead with hands until well mixed. Use flour on hands and kneading surface to keep the mixture from sticking. Continue to add flour to alleviate stickiness as necessary.

EXERCISE 14 • Memorizing Major Muscle Information

There are many ways to organize, review, and memorize the specific origins, insertions, and actions of the muscles. Many learners make or buy flash cards (for suggestions on how to make and use flash cards, see Chapter 2, Exercise 1), while others use mind maps or tables. For example, the two tables shown here organize the muscles by joint and list their actions before their origins and insertions. This organizational focus on function may be particularly helpful for kinesthetic learners who relate to action over origin and insertion. Notice that the primary functions are in bold, while secondary or assistive functions are in normal type. In addition, if you highlight each function with a different color, you will easily be able to identify all the muscles that contribute to a specific joint movement. The scapulothoracic table is highlighted for you.

Scapulothoracic Articulation

MUSCLE	ACTION(S)	ORIGIN	INSERTION
Trapezius 3 portions— upper, mid, lower	**Elevation** (upper) **Retraction** (mid) **Depression** (lower) Upward rotation of the scapula (upper; lower)	Occiput, nuchal ligament, and spinous processes of C7–T12	Lateral one-third of clavicle, acromion process and full spine of the scapula
Levator scapula	**Elevation** **Downward rotation** of the scapula	Transverse processes of C1–C4	Superior angle to the root of the scapular spine
Rhomboids	**Retraction** Downward rotation of the scapula	Spinous processes of C7–T5	Medial border of the scapula
Serratus anterior	**Protraction** **Upward rotation** of the scapula **Stabilization** of the scapula during shoulder movement	Anterolateral ribs 1–8	Vertebral border of the scapula
Pectoralis minor	**Protraction** **Depression** Downward rotation of the scapula	Anterior surface of ribs 3–5	Coracoid process
Subclavius	**Depression** of the clavicle **Stabilization** of the sternoclavicular joint	First rib	Inferior edge of the clavicle

Elevation: upper trap, levator scap; **Retraction:** mid trap, rhomboids; **Upward rotation:** upper and lower trap, serratus.
Depression: L trap, pec minor, **Protraction:** serratus, pec minor; **Downward rotation:** levator, rhomboids, pec minor.

If this technique is useful, go ahead and add your own highlights to the elbow table.

Elbow (Humeroulnar) and Radioulnar Joints

MUSCLE	ACTION(S)	ORIGIN	INSERTION
Biceps brachii	**Flexion** **Supination** Assists in shoulder flexion	Coracoid process and supraglenoid tubercle	Radial tuberosity
Brachialis	**Flexion**	Anterior distal half of the humerus	Coronoid process and ulnar tuberosity
Brachioradialis	**Flexion**	Lateral supracondylar ridge of the humerus	Styloid process of the radius
Triceps brachii	**Extension** Assists in shoulder extension	Infraglenoid tubercle, proximal posterior and distal shaft of the humerus	Olecranon process
Anconeus	**Extension**	Lateral epicondyle of the humerus	Olecranon process
Pronator teres	**Pronation**	Medial epicondyle of the humerus	Mid-lateral shaft of the radius
Pronator quadratus	**Pronation**	Distal anterior ulna	Distal anterior radius
Supinator	**Supination**	Lateral epicondyle of the humerus and posterior proximal ulna	Proximal lateral shaft of the radius

Humeroulnar joint motions: Flexion—biceps brachii, brachialis, brachioradialis; **Extension**—triceps brachii, anconeus.
Radioulnar joint motions: Supination—biceps brachii, supinator; **Pronation**—pronator teres, pronator quadratus.

6: The Skeletal Muscle System

REVIEW QUIZ

Skeletal Muscle System

Multiple Choice: Select the one best answer.

1. What are the functions of the skeletal muscle system?
   A. generate heat, protect vital organs, coordinate movement, and store energy
   B. create movement, help stabilize joints, maintain posture, and generate heat
   C. help stabilize joints and maintain body temperature, plus coordinate the muscular and skeletal systems during movement
   D. maintain our upright position, store energy and proteins, generate movement and heat

2. The key characteristics that describe the functional qualities of skeletal muscles are excitable, contractile _____, and _____.
   A. elastic; resilient
   B. tough; fibrous
   C. extensible; elastic
   D. resilient; cylindrical

3. Two muscles that attach to bone via an aponeurosis rather than a tendon are
   A. tensor fasciae latae and gastrocnemius.
   B. transverse abdominis and pectineus.
   C. latissimus dorsi and iliocostalis.
   D. quadratus lumborum and pectoralis major.

4. Which of these is the best explanation of the all-or-none principle of muscle contraction?
   A. All fibers in a motor unit must contract fully when sufficient stimulus is delivered.
   B. All motor units in a muscle will contract when threshold stimulus is delivered.
   C. Muscle fibers must contract fully when all stimulus is delivered.
   D. No muscle fibers in the unit contract until all motor neurons are stimulated.

5. The sliding filament theory explains that muscle fibers contract when _____ is released from the sarcoplasmic reticulum, causing the myofilaments to bond and slide over each other.
   A. calcium
   B. potassium
   C. neurotransmitter
   D. nitrogen

6. What is the smallest contractile unit of a muscle?
   A. fascicle
   B. motor unit
   C. muscle fiber
   D. sarcomere

7. What is the name for the large grouping of muscle fibers surrounded by the perimysium?
   A. the belly
   B. muscle compartment
   C. fascicle
   D. myofibrils

8. Which of these tissue characteristics is true of fascia?
   A. densely packed fibers
   B. low ratio of elastic and reticular fibers
   C. highly organized parallel arrangement of fibers
   D. lots of ground substance that keeps fibers widely spaced

9. A motor unit is composed of one motor neuron and
   A. a single muscle fiber.
   B. multiple muscle fibers.
   C. two fascicles.
   D. several sarcomeres.

10. The graded response theory explains how the force of muscle contraction is changed by
    A. increasing or decreasing the number of motor units stimulated.
    B. increasing the amount of calcium released into the sarcomere.
    C. altering the amount of stimulus applied to the muscle.
    D. shifting the role of the muscle from agonist to synergist.

11. What is the term used to describe the minimum amount of stimulus required for muscle contraction?
    A. minimum stimulus
    B. contractile stimulus
    C. threshold stimulus
    D. tetanic stimulus

80 REVIEW GUIDE

12. Which method of energy production for muscle contraction provides the quick energy needed for short bursts of activity?
   A. aerobic glycolysis
   B. anaerobic cellular metabolism
   C. aerobic cellular metabolism
   D. direct phosphorylation (ATP-CP)

13. Which method of energy production for muscle contraction creates lactic acid and the largest oxygen debt?
   A. direct phosphorylation
   B. anaerobic cellular metabolism
   C. aerobic cellular metabolism
   D. Krebs cycle

14. What type of muscle contraction maintains our posture and each muscle's state of readiness for contraction?
   A. isometric
   B. tonic
   C. concentric
   D. tetanic

15. A muscle contraction that radically increases the tension in the muscle but does not result in movement of a body part is classified as
   A. tonic.
   B. isotonic.
   C. eccentric.
   D. isometric.

16. The pectoralis major and biceps brachii are both examples of _____ fiber arrangements.
   A. fusiform
   B. bipennate
   C. triangular
   D. parallel

17. What movement role is assigned to an antagonist muscle?
   A. oppose the primary movement
   B. create the primary movement
   C. assist in creating the primary movement
   D. stabilize an adjacent bone during movement

18. What is the name for the muscle attachment that is generally fixed or stabilized during movement?
   A. insertion
   B. fixed attachment
   C. origin
   D. primary attachment

19. What term is used to describe the natural state of firmness of a muscle due to the status of the tissue and fluid elements?
   A. motor tone
   B. muscle tonicity
   C. muscle tone
   D. muscle spasm

20. What type of contraction occurs when a muscle is functioning as the prime mover?
   A. concentric isotonic
   B. tonic
   C. isometric
   D. eccentric isotonic

21. Which category of ROM is best for assessing the available range of movement and the status of the inert tissues around a joint?
   A. active
   B. assistive
   C. passive
   D. resistive

22. What is the primary function of the quadriceps muscle group?
   A. hip extension
   B. knee extension
   C. knee flexion
   D. hip extension

23. The three muscles that are prime movers in elbow flexion are the biceps brachii, brachioradialis, and
   A. coracobrachialis.
   B. brachialis.
   C. triceps brachii.
   D. flexor carpi radialis.

24. The "rotator cuff" muscles that move the humerus include the supraspinatus, infraspinatus, subscapularis, and
   A. teres major.
   B. deltoid.
   C. rhomboids.
   D. teres minor.

25. What muscle in the hip adductor group also flexes the knee?
   A. pectineus
   B. adductor longus
   C. gracilis
   D. adductor magnus

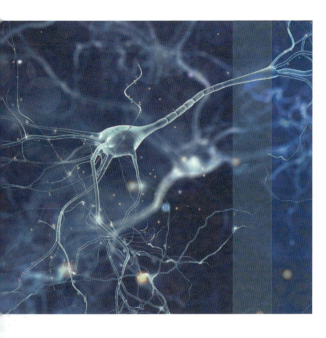

7

The Nervous System

Use this list to choose learning exercises that will help you expand and solidify your understanding of key topics. To test your knowledge, try the Review Quiz at the end of the chapter.

Key Topics	Exercise
• System Terminology	1 & 11
• Organization of the System	2
• Neurons and Neuroglia	3–5
• Nerve Structure	6
• Impulse Conduction	7
• Sensory Receptors	9
• CNS Coverings	10
• The Spinal Cord	11, 12, 18
• The Brain	13–15
• Neuronal Pathways	8, 15, 16
• The ANS	17

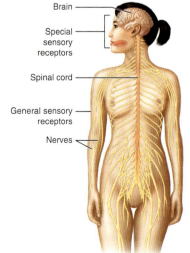

EXERCISE 1 • Nervous System Crossword

Use this crossword to review and test your knowledge of some of the nervous system's structures and functions.

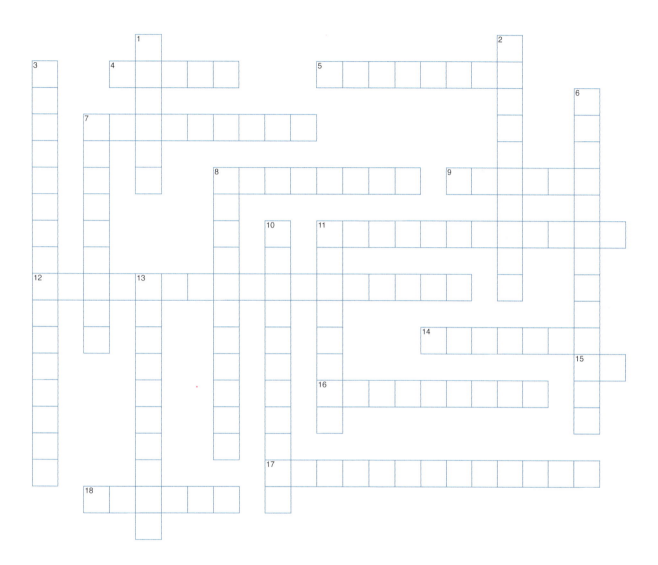

ACROSS

4 Parasympathetic cranial nerve that innervates the viscera.
5 Meningeal layer that supports the large blood vessels on the surface of the brain and spinal cord.
7 Tough outermost meningeal layer.
8 Nerve plexus that innervates the head and neck.
9 Nerve plexus that consists of L1 through L4 spinal nerves.
11 Specific gray matter motor regions of the cerebrum.
12 Boundary that protects brain from pathogens present in blood.
14 Muscle(s) innervated by a specific spinal nerve and cord segment.
15 The number for the accessory cranial nerve.
16 Meningeal layer where cerebral spinal fluid circulates.
17 Colorless fluid that cushions and nourishes the structures of the CNS.
18 Cranial nerve affected by Bell's palsy.

DOWN

1 Nerve plexus whose branches include the sciatic nerve.
2 Cranial nerve V.
3 The brain stem region that contains the respiratory rhythmicity and cardiovascular centers.
6 Specialized capillaries lined with ependymal neuroglia that produce CSF.
7 Area of skin innervated by sensory fibers from a specific spinal nerve and cord segment.
8 Horse's tail of the spinal cord.
10 A neural circuit in which several neurons synapse on a single neuron.
11 Nerve plexus whose branches include the axillary, radial, and ulnar nerves.
13 A neural circuit in which one neuron synapses with several neurons.

EXERCISE 2 • Functional Organization of the Nervous System

Under the umbrella of the nervous system, there are two major divisions. Fill in all of the components of the system below, starting with the two major divisions (boxes 1 and 2). Then use blue to color the divisions and structures responsible for sensory functions, green for integrative functions, and red for motor functions. If you need to refresh your memory, refer to Figures 7.1 and 7.28 in your textbook.

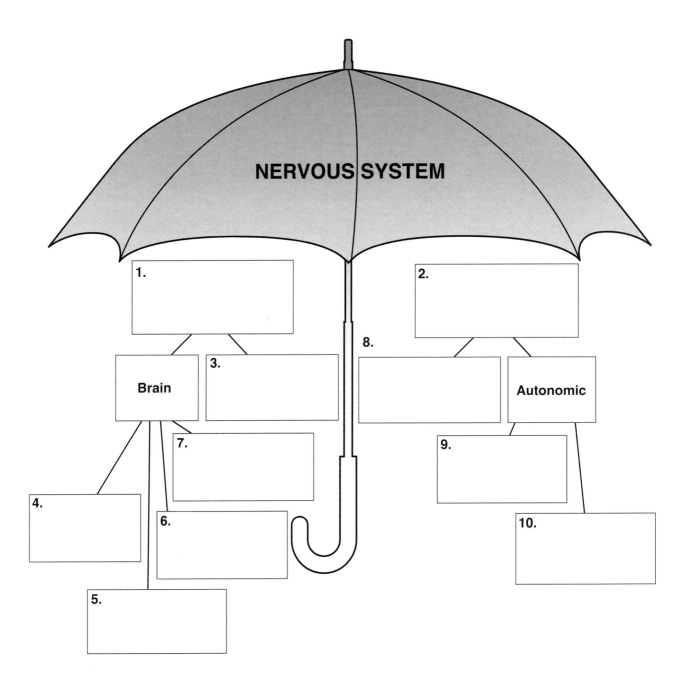

EXERCISE 3 • Neuroglia Mind Map

Complete the mind map by filling in the names and functions of the six types of neuroglia.
Color the neuroglia found in the CNS green and those found in the PNS purple.

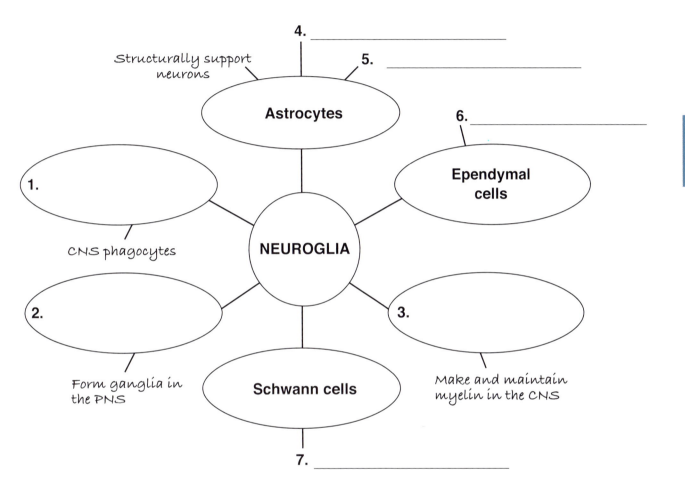

EXERCISE 4 • Matching Neuron Parts

Complete the matching exercise by placing the letter of the answer that best matches the term provided.

_____ **1.** Axon

_____ **2.** Axon hillock

_____ **3.** Axon terminal

_____ **4.** Myelin

_____ **5.** Cell body

_____ **6.** Dendrites

_____ **7.** Nucleus

_____ **8.** Sensory neuron

_____ **9.** Interneuron

_____ **10.** Motor neuron

_____ **11.** Unipolar

_____ **12.** Bipolar

_____ **13.** Multipolar

_____ **14.** Neurilemma

_____ **15.** Synaptic bulb

A. Location of the synaptic bulbs

B. Carries impulses to the CNS

C. Carries impulses to effectors

D. Transmits impulse away from the cell body

E. Transmit impulse toward the cell body

F. Plasma membrane of a Schwann cell

G. Location of the neuron's nucleus

H. Many dendrites and one axon

I. Contains vesicles with neurotransmitters

J. Region where an action potential is generated

K. Cell body between one dendrite and one axon

L. Location of DNA

M. One fiber with a cell body off to one side

N. Insulating sheath of fat

O. Found only in the CNS

EXERCISE 5 • Neurons and Their Parts

Label the neuron diagrams. The terms in the matching exercise may provide you with clues, or if you need to refresh your memory, refer to Figures 7.2 and 7.3 in your textbook.

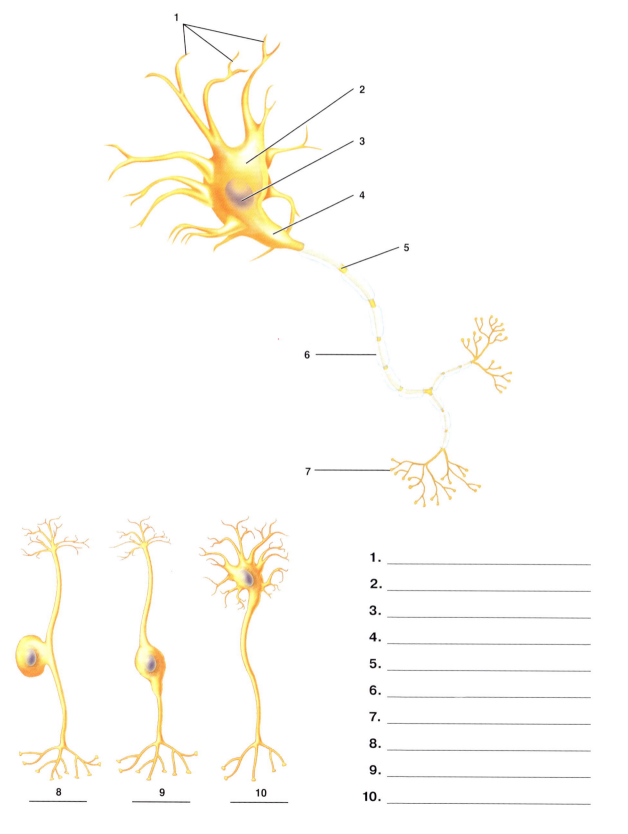

1. _____
2. _____
3. _____
4. _____
5. _____
6. _____
7. _____
8. _____
9. _____
10. _____

7: The Nervous System   87

EXERCISE 6 • Structure of a Nerve

A nerve is a bundle of axons with its connective tissue coverings and blood vessels outside the CNS. There are _____ pairs of _____ nerves exiting the underside of the brain, and _____ pairs of _____ nerves that relate to the segments of the spinal cord.

Color and label the parts of a nerve on the diagram below. If you need to refresh your memory, refer to Figure 7.5 in your textbook.

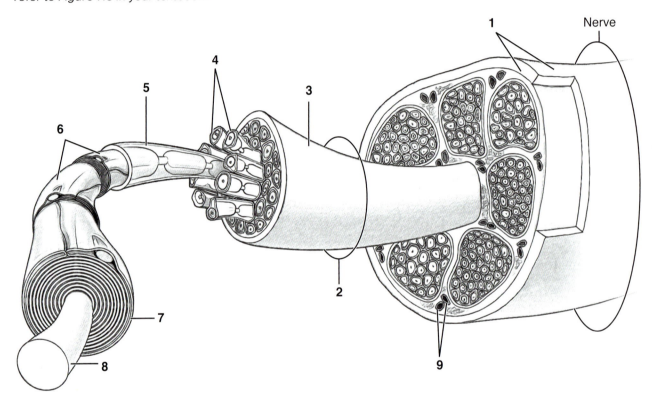

1. _____
2. _____
3. _____
4. _____
5. _____
6. _____
7. _____
8. _____
9. _____

88   REVIEW GUIDE

EXERCISE 7 • A Story of Impulse Conduction

Taking the steps of a physiologic process and turning them into a story can help with understanding and recall. The following provides one example of how a story about the key steps of nerve impulse conduction and synaptic transmission might begin. Have fun completing this story or write a different story altogether.

Once upon a time, a traveler named "Impulse" entered the tiny hamlet of Neurolandia and traveled down the main street named Neuron Avenue. Because of his rather gloomy and negative attitude, Impulse created change wherever he walked. . . .

EXERCISE 8 • Diagram a Reflex Arc

Reflexes are automatic and involuntary responses that require little interpretation by the integrating center. A reflex arc is a simple neuronal pathway that provides a predictable motor **1.** _____ for a specific sensory **2.** _____. Deep tendon reflexes are managed by **3.** _____ _____ reflex arcs, while the withdrawal reflex is an example of a **4.** _____ _____ reflex arc.

Color and label the components of the reflex arcs diagrammed below, making any sensory components blue, integrative components green, and motor components red. If you need to refresh your memory, refer to Figure 7.14 in your textbook.

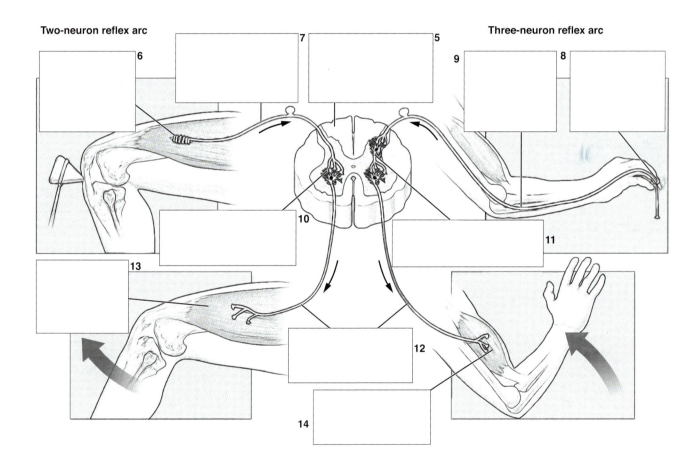

EXERCISE 9 • Sensory Receptors Table

Fill in the blanks to complete this table describing the different categories of sensory receptors, the stimulus each is sensitive to, and example(s) of the location for each category.

RECEPTOR CATEGORY	STIMULUS	EXAMPLE LOCATION
1.	Light	2.
NOCICEPTORS	3.	4.
5.	6.	Joints and skeletal muscles
MECHANORECEPTORS	7.	8.
9.	Changes in chemical concentrations	10.
THERMORECEPTORS	11.	12.

EXERCISE 10 • Meninges Diagram

Label the diagram of the meninges covering the brain. If you need to refresh your memory, refer to Figure 7.20 in your textbook.

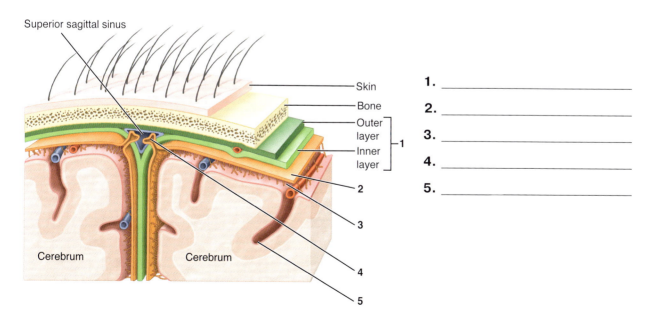

1. _____
2. _____
3. _____
4. _____
5. _____

EXERCISE 11 • Nervous Terminology: Reviewing Synonyms

In the nervous system, structures are referred to by a variety of synonymous terms. For example, sensory neurons can also be referred to as **1.** _____ neurons because they transmit impulses toward the CNS, while **2.** _____ neurons are often called efferent neurons because they transmit impulses away from the CNS. Other structures that have several synonymous names include the spinal cord tracts and the nerve roots that split apart from the spinal nerves to attach to the cord.

Use the diagram below to name the tracts and nerve roots. Place your preferred name on the line within the box and identify synonyms next to the bullets.

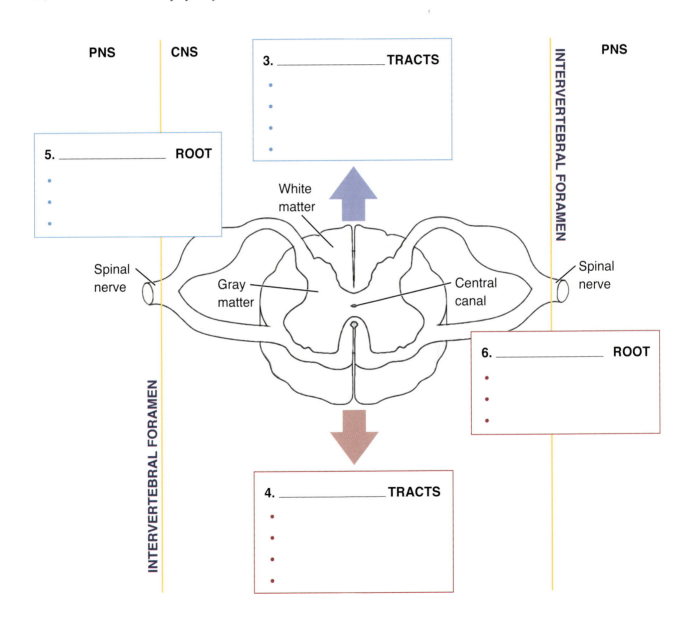

92 REVIEW GUIDE

EXERCISE 12 • Spinal Cord Gray Matter Organization

The gray matter of the spinal cord is divided into three major regions, or horns. The posterior horn receives sensory information, while the lateral and anterior horns contain the cell bodies and dendrites of motor neurons.

Color and label the four regions designated on the right side of the diagram to identify what information is received or sent from each region. Label the horns on the left side. If you need to refresh your memory, refer to Figure 7.22 in your textbook.

1 gray horn

2 gray horn

3 gray horn

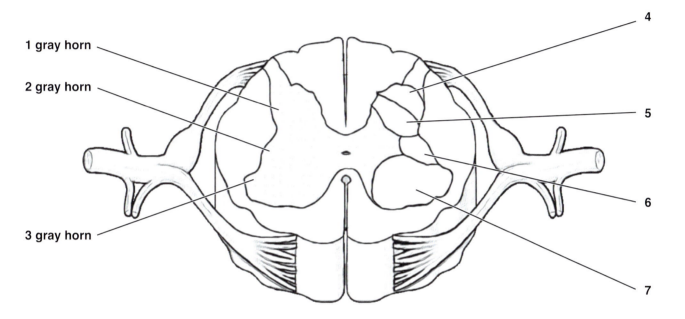

1. _____
2. _____
3. _____
4. _____
5. _____
6. _____
7. _____

EXERCISE 13 • Matching Brain Parts and Their Functions

Color and label the parts of the brain identified on the diagram. Then, using the list provided, place the letter that best describes the function of each region next to its name. If you need to refresh your memory, refer to Figure 7.24 and the sections about the various brain regions in your textbook.

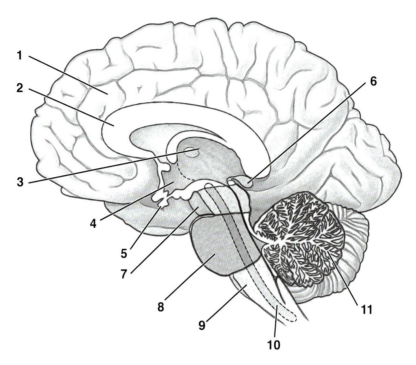

1. _____
2. _____
3. _____
4. _____
5. _____
6. _____
7. _____
8. _____
9. _____
10. _____
11. _____

A. Serves as a sensory clearing house

B. Controls reflexes including coughing, sneezing, and swallowing and contains the respiratory rhythmicity and cardiovascular centers

C. A white matter bridge that allows information to be shared between the cerebral hemispheres

D. Releases hormones that control other endocrine glands

E. Controls and coordinates muscle contractions for body movement, posture, and balance

F. Controls the ANS and links the nervous and endocrine systems

G. Manages conscious thought, creative thinking, and other complex processes

H. Forms important connections between the spinal cord, cerebellum, and cerebrum

I. Helps to coordinate muscle contractions and controls movements of the eyes, head, and neck in response to visual stimuli

J. Manages state of alertness and helps regulate resting muscle tone, digestion, urination, and sexual arousal

K. Secretes melatonin

EXERCISE 14 • Cerebral Structures

The cerebral cortex that covers the white matter of the cerebrum is characterized by its many folds, or
1. _____. Deep **2.** _____ (1 and 2 on the diagram) divide the cerebrum into two
3. _____ (3 and 4 on the diagram). Shallow grooves called **4.** _____ (5 and 6)
divide each half into four **5.** _____ (7 through 10).

Label the diagram below to identify the location of these structures. If you need to refresh your memory, refer to Figure 7.25 in your textbook.

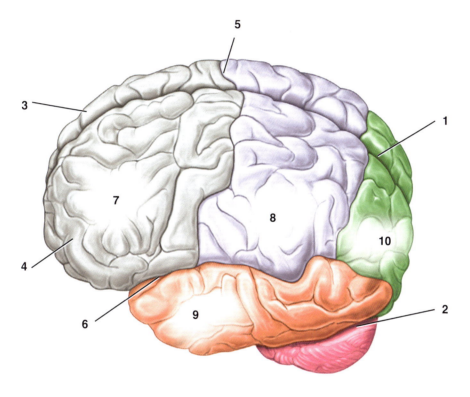

1. _____
2. _____
3. _____
4. _____
5. _____
6. _____
7. _____
8. _____
9. _____
10. _____

EXERCISE 15 • Pathways of the Nervous System

The CNS interprets and processes sensory information from the PNS and coordinates and controls motor commands to effectors. Neurons carrying sensory information form afferent pathways, while neurons transmitting motor information form efferent pathways.

Place the number or letter from the diagram that matches each of the structures in the list below. (Hint: the arrows show the direction impulses are traveling.) Then, color the afferent pathways on the diagram blue and the efferent pathways red. If you choose, color the structures of the CNS and/or add more colors to distinguish the different types of PNS motor neurons on the diagram.

Neurons and tracts (letters)

_____ Sensory neurons

_____ Somatic motor neurons

_____ Sympathetic motor neurons

_____ Parasympathetic motor neurons

_____ Ascending tracts

_____ Descending tracts

Brain and cord (numbers)

_____ Spinal cord

_____ Cauda equina

_____ Cerebrum

_____ Diencephalon

_____ Brain stem

_____ Cerebellum

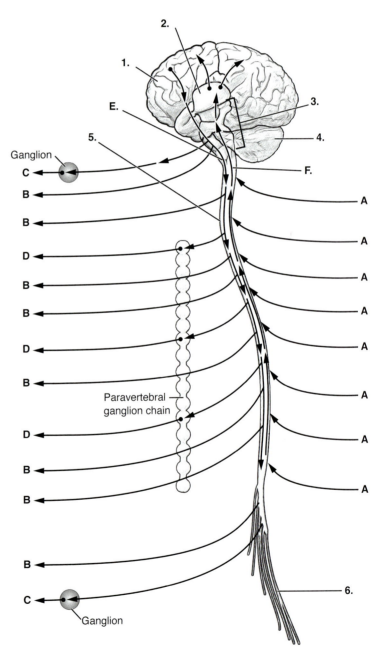

96 REVIEW GUIDE

EXERCISE 16 • Comparing Somatic and Autonomic Motor Pathways

Use the Venn diagram below to compare and contrast the structural and functional characteristics of somatic and autonomic pathways. An example of one shared characteristic—that is, include sensory and motor neurons—has been placed in the area of overlap to get you started. Other characteristics to consider might include number of motor neurons in the divisions' pathways, types of effectors, neurotransmitters used by motor neurons, or nerves carrying the motor pathways (specific cranial or spinal nerves). If you need to review how to use a Venn diagram, refer to Chapter 6, Exercise 3.

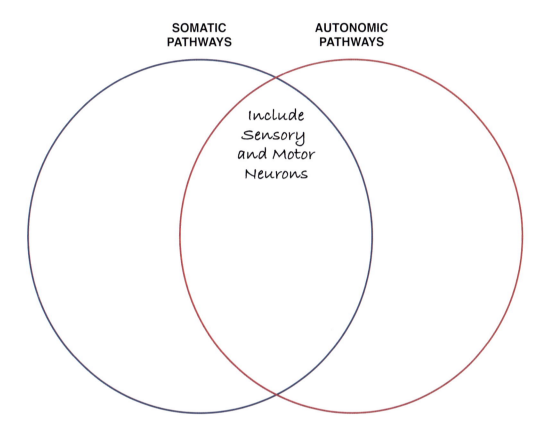

EXERCISE 17 • ANS Features

Complete the following table that compares and contrasts the features and functions of the two branches of the ANS.

CHARACTERISTIC	SYMPATHETIC	PARASYMPATHETIC
Nickname for division based on general function or effect	1.	2.
Name of division based on nerves that carry the ANS motor pathways	3.	4.
Number of motor neurons in each ANS pathway	5.	6.
Location of ganglia	7.	8.
Widespread or targeted stimulation of effectors	9.	10.
Neurotransmitter released by the postganglionic neurons	11.	12.

7: The Nervous System

EXERCISE 18 • Building a Model of the Spinal Cord

To better understand the structure of the spinal cord, you can build a simple 3D model using materials easily obtained from any craft store. While you can do this activity alone, it is often more helpful to do it with a group of people. Each person in your group will build a single cord segment. Then you can stack these segments together to form a portion of the spinal cord. For each segment, you will need:

One 3- to 4-inch round disk of styrofoam, white clay, or white cardboard that is approximately 1 inch thick

Gray-colored felt or paper

Six blue pipe cleaners

Six red pipe cleaners

Glue

Clear plastic wrap or tape

Follow these steps to create your model. You may find it helpful to refer to Figure 7.22A in your textbook.

1. Draw and cut a butterfly shape out of the gray-colored felt or paper to represent the gray matter of the spinal cord (don't forget the central canal). Glue it to the top of your disk to create a spinal cord segment. Once the gray matter is in place, be sure everyone in your group is clear where the anterior and posterior regions of their segment are located.

2. Using the blue pipe cleaners to represent sensory neurons, insert three sensory neurons on each side of the segment adjacent to the proper horn of gray matter. Twist a small loop in the pipe cleaners to represent the dorsal root ganglion.

3. Using the red pipe cleaners to represent motor neurons, insert three motor neurons on each side of the segment adjacent to the proper horn of gray matter.

4. Bring the three sensory neurons and three motor neurons on each side together to form a spinal nerve on either side of your spinal cord segment. Wrap your spinal nerve together with your plastic wrap or tape. Notice how the nerve divides close to the cord into dorsal and ventral roots.

5. Finally, stack your segments together to create a portion of the spinal cord. Be sure all your sensory neurons (blues) are on the dorsal side and the motor neurons (reds) are on the ventral side.

REVIEW QUIZ

The Nervous System

Multiple Choice: Select the one best answer.

1. Three primary messaging functions of the nervous system are sensory,_____, and _____.
   A. motor; autonomic
   B. sympathetic; parasympathetic
   C. integration; motor
   D. cognitive; coordination

2. What are the three types or classifications of neurons by function?
   A. bipolar, unipolar, and polypolar
   B. associative, sensory, and motor
   C. afferent, associative, and interneuron
   D. sensory, autonomic, and motor

3. Which of these glial cells produce myelin in the central nervous system?
   A. astrocytes
   B. Schwann cells
   C. microglia
   D. oligodendrocytes

4. What are the four regions of the brain?
   A. brain stem, cerebrum, diencephalon, cerebellum
   B. cerebellum, thalamus, hypothalamus, cerebrum
   C. medulla oblongata, cerebrum, cerebellum, corpus collosum
   D. cerebrum, parietal, occipital, temporal

5. What is the name of cranial nerve V?
   A. facial
   B. trigeminal
   C. vagus
   D. optic

6. The C8 nerve is positioned between which vertebrae?
   A. C-6 and C-7
   B. T-1 and T-2
   C. C-7 and T-1
   D. C-8 and T-1

7. Which spinal nerve plexus innervates the upper extremity?
   A. brachial
   B. cervical
   C. thoracic
   D. lumbar

8. Major nerve branches off the lumbar plexus include the ilioinguinal, obturator, _____, and _____.
   A. peroneal; tibial
   B. sciatic; femoral
   C. femoral; lateral femoral cutaneous
   D. greater saphenous; lesser saphenous

9. Which region of the brain is responsible for coordinating voluntary muscles and maintaining posture?
   A. cerebrum
   B. pons
   C. medulla oblongata
   D. cerebellum

10. What is another term for a nerve impulse?
    A. polarization
    B. action potential
    C. threshold stimulus
    D. depolarization

11. What forms the chemical bridge that acts as a stimulus for an effector or postsynaptic neuron?
    A. neurotransmitters
    B. sodium ions
    C. neurolemma
    D. repolarized ions

12. When one neuron stimulates an entire group of postsynaptic neurons, it is an example of what type of neuronal circuit?
    A. postsynaptic pool
    B. convergence
    C. divergence
    D. neural spray

13. Which of the following is an example of a somatic effector?
    A. heart
    B. stomach
    C. blood vessels
    D. biceps femoris

14. Which of the special sense receptors are examples of chemoreceptors?
    A. taste and smell
    B. pressure and auditory
    C. vision and equilibrium
    D. taste and vision

7: The Nervous System

15. What type and combination of neurons make up the sympathetic and parasympathetic pathways?
    A. one sensory and one motor
    B. one each of sensory, motor, and associative
    C. one associative and one motor
    D. two motor neurons

16. Muscle spindles are most sensitive to what type of stimulus?
    A. sudden shortening
    B. rapid lengthening
    C. slow lengthening
    D. alternating short-long

17. Which of the following terms are synonymous to sensory tracts?
    A. descending and ventral tracts
    B. ventral and anterior tracts
    C. lateral and visceral tracts
    D. ascending and dorsal tracts

18. Cerebrospinal fluid circulates in what layer of the meninges?
    A. dura mater
    B. arachnoid
    C. pia mater
    D. subdural space

19. The functions of cerebrospinal fluid are to act as a shock absorber, create a physical barrier between blood and brain, and
    A. act as the medium for nutrient waste exchange.
    B. carry out all immune processes in CNS.
    C. provide lubrication to the brain and cranial nerves.
    D. serve as the primary neurotransmitter for brain and spinal cord.

20. What kind of dysfunction is most likely to occur when the anterior root of a spinal nerve is damaged?
    A. full loss of sensation in the associated dermatome
    B. partial loss of sensation in a few dermatomes
    C. loss of movement and/or muscle strength
    D. paresthesia and decreased smooth muscle function

21. What part of the brain stem serves as the center for the cardiac, respiratory, and vascular motor reflexes?
    A. midbrain
    B. hypothalamus
    C. pons
    D. medulla oblongata

22. Virtually all sensory information is sorted, prioritized, and routed through which structure in the brain?
    A. hypothalamus
    B. thalamus
    C. medulla oblongata
    D. pineal gland

23. What is the function of the corpus callosum?
    A. produce cerebrospinal fluid
    B. relay information between cerebellum and cerebrum
    C. junction between the two cerebral hemispheres
    D. center for emotions like anger, fear, and anxiety

24. Which region of the brain is known as the "emotional brain"?
    A. cerebral cortex
    B. corpus callosum
    C. hypothalamus
    D. limbic system

25. Which CNS structure is the control center for the autonomic functions of the nervous system?
    A. cerebellum
    B. hypothalamus
    C. thalamus
    D. medulla oblongata

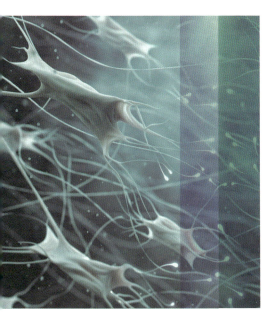

8

Neuromuscular and Myofascial Connections

Use this list to choose learning exercises that will help you expand and solidify your understanding of key topics. To test your knowledge, try the Review Quiz at the end of the chapter.

Key Topics	Exercise
• Terminology	1
• Neuromuscular Reflexes and Loops	2 & 3
• Trigger and Tender Points	4
• Tensegrity	5
• Fascial Layers and Planes	6
• Mechanical Properties of Fascia	7
• Fascial Receptors	8
• Posture, Balance, and Coordinated Movement	9

EXERCISE 1 • Neuromuscular and Myofascial Terminology Crossword

Use this crossword to review and test your knowledge of the anatomy and physiology terms from Chapter 8.

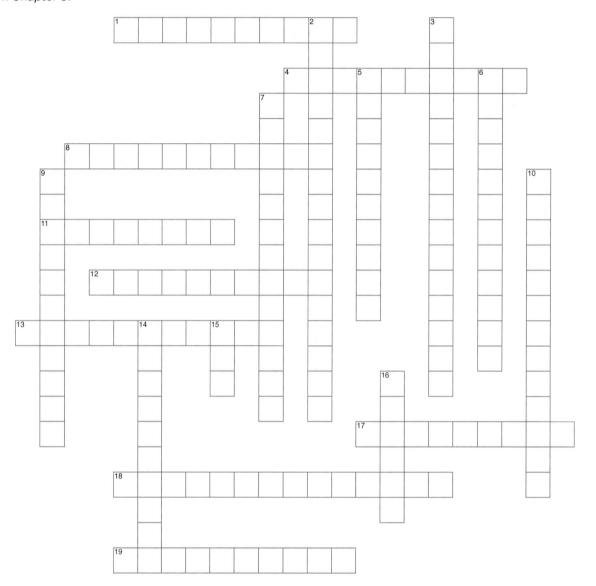

ACROSS

1. The ability of a substance to vacillate between gel and sol states.
4. Connective tissue layers that organize and surround individual muscles, bones, and organs; the axial, visceral, and meningeal layers.
8. Low-grade tension created by smooth muscle cells within fascia that is regulated by the ANS.
11. Skeletal muscles that play an essential role in maintaining the body's upright position are called _____.
12. The superficial layer or tube of fascia.
13. The sense and awareness of movement.
17. Pretensioning of the muscle spindle that increases its sensitivity to rapid lengthening.
18. Sense and awareness of where body parts are positioned in space and in relationship to one another.
19. A very powerful GAG; _____ acid.

DOWN

2. Small electrical charge along a cell or tissue surface created by mechanical pressure.
3. The ability of tissues to extend and rebound rather than to stretch and recoil.
5. The ability of a substance to be molded or changed.
6. Most abundant myofascial sensory receptors.
7. Triple helix protein molecule found in collagen fibers.
9. Hypodermis is also known as the _____ fascia.
10. Excessive muscle tension.
14. System in which tension between two opposing forces is balanced to create structural integrity.
15. A more liquid state.
16. Skeletal muscles whose primary role is to create movement are called _____.

EXERCISE 2 • Neuromuscular Reflexes Table

This table will help you organize the information about different neuromuscular reflexes and their implications for manual therapy. Simply place the letter of the muscle reflex definitions and manual therapy applications into the proper row and column to fill in the table. One manual therapy application has already been provided.

Definitions

A. The alpha neuronal pathway of muscle spindles is stimulated by lengthening or stretching of the extrafusal fibers and signals a reflexive contraction of the muscle.

B. The reflex mechanism that coordinates the effort between agonist and antagonist muscles. Reciprocal innervation (RI) between agonist and antagonist gives a simultaneous motor command for the agonist to contract and inhibition of contraction in the antagonist.

C. The gamma neuronal pathway of muscle spindles becomes hypersensitive to the rate of lengthening so that sudden lengthening of a muscle creates a "false stretch reflex" report that locks the muscle into a slightly shortened position. This response is especially pronounced if a muscle has been static or shortened for a period of time prior to rapid lengthening.

D. Golgi tendon organs that are sensitive to tension within skeletal muscle respond to the increased tension of an active muscle contraction by inhibiting its force.

Manual Therapy Application

E. Therapists employ a contract-relax method to a tight muscle that inhibits muscle tension to enhance stretch and gain improved range.

F. Therapists can reduce tension in tight muscles by engaging the antagonist of that muscle in an isometric contraction because it causes contraction of the tight muscle to be inhibited.

G. Static stretching (slow and gradual) is used to improve muscle length and ROM because it avoids stimulating a stretch reflex (SR) and possible tissue damage.

TYPE OF MUSCLE REFLEX	DEFINITION	MANUAL THERAPY APPLICATION
Stretch reflex	1.	2.
Gamma gain	3.	By shortening a muscle with TeP, and holding that position for approximately 90 seconds, therapists turn off the false SR report. Therapists must slowly and passively move the muscle back to normal resting length to avoid restimulation of the contraction.
Inverse stretch reflex	4.	5.
Reciprocal innervation	6.	7.

8: Neuromuscular and Myofascial Connections

EXERCISE 3 • Neuronal Loops

Complete the fill-in-the-blank exercise and then color the diagram to identify the two types of muscle fibers and the neurons of the neuronal pathways associated with muscle spindles. Notice that the numbers in the diagram match the numbers in the fill-in-the-blank exercise and colors for the different neurons are suggested. If you need to refresh your memory, refer to Figure 8.2 and the sections on neuromuscular reflexes in your textbook.

Muscle spindles are proprioceptors that sense **1.** _____ of muscle

fibers and signal a reflexive **2.** _____ of the muscle called the

3. _____ _____. Muscle spindles have two distinct

portions linked to different neuronal pathways that innervate different types of muscle fibers. The alpha

loop is made up of the **4.** _____ _____ neuron

(blue) looped around the central region of the muscle spindle and the **5.** _____

_____ neuron **(red)** that innervates **6.** _____

fibers within the muscle. The alpha loop is the reflex arc for the **7.** _____

_____. In addition, the alpha neurons are also part of the sensory

and motor pathways used by the primary motor centers of the cerebrum and cerebellum to

8. _____.

The second reflex arc, called the **9.** _____ _____,

is composed of a **10.** _____ _____ neuron

(purple) attached toward the ends of the spindle and the **11.** _____

_____ neuron **(orange)** that innervates the **12.** _____

fibers. This reflex arc regulates the **13.** _____ of the muscle spindle by

adjusting its **14.** _____ and _____ In other words,

when stimulated to contract via this neuronal loop, the **15.** _____ within the

muscle spindle increases, effectively increasing the proprioceptor's **16.** _____

to any lengthening of the muscle. This phenomenon is called **17.** _____

_____.

104   REVIEW GUIDE

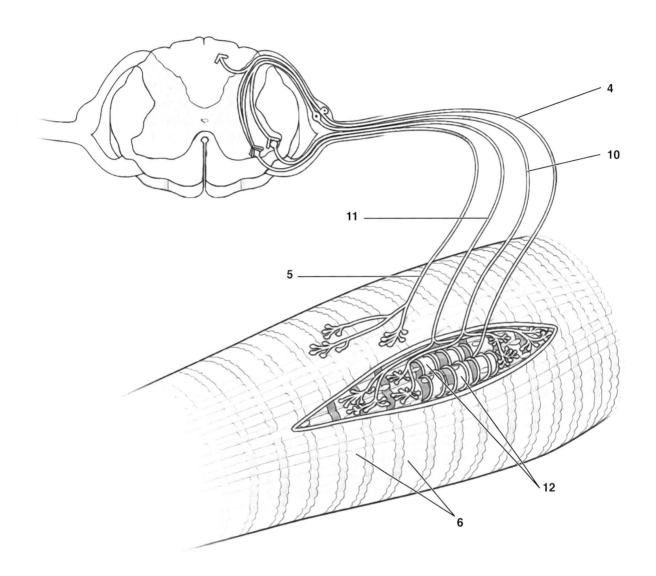

EXERCISE 4 • Trigger Versus Tender Points

Identify each statement below as characteristic of trigger points (TP), tender points (TeP), or both (B).

_____ **1.** Point is often not palpable

_____ **2.** Point is hypersensitive to mechanical pressure

_____ **3.** Caused by high gamma gain in the muscle spindle

_____ **4.** Has a palpable nodule in a taut band of muscle

_____ **5.** Digital pressure reproduces pain complaint in a predictable pattern

_____ **6.** Caused by chemical irritation of motor end plate

_____ **7.** Stretching can recreate the pain at this point

_____ **8.** Digital pressure creates no referred pattern of pain

_____ **9.** Muscles with this point are resistant to full stretch

_____ **10.** "Calcium spill" into sarcomere leads to actin-myosin bonding

_____ **11.** Often silent until compressed

_____ **12.** Treatment requires repositioning of muscle

EXERCISE 5 • Tensegrity

The term tensegrity describes how the **1.** _____ between two opposing forces can be balanced to create structural **2.** _____. In the musculoskeletal system, gravity creates a **3.** _____ force on the bones of the skeleton, while the muscles and fascia that connect and functionally integrate the skeleton exert **4.** _____ on the bones and joints to maintain **5.** _____ _____

The musculoskeletal system is not the only example of tensegrity in the human body. For example, the functional integrity of the nervous system relies on both convergent and divergent pathways. Convergent pathways allow for a single control decision to be made from multiple pieces of information, while divergent pathways allow many regions of the brain or effectors to respond to a singular piece of information. What other examples of tensegrity can you think of in the human body or in your life?

EXERCISE 6 • Fascial Layers and Planes

Use the lists provided to label and identify the different layers, bands, and planes of fascia by color in each of the diagrams. If you need to refresh your memory, refer to Figures 8.7 and 8.11 in your textbook.

Fascial Layers

Each layer of fascia creates a tube or organizing sleeve for its structures. All four sleeves merge together at the **1.** _____ _____

- Axial layer
- Meningeal layer
- Pannicular layer
- Visceral layer

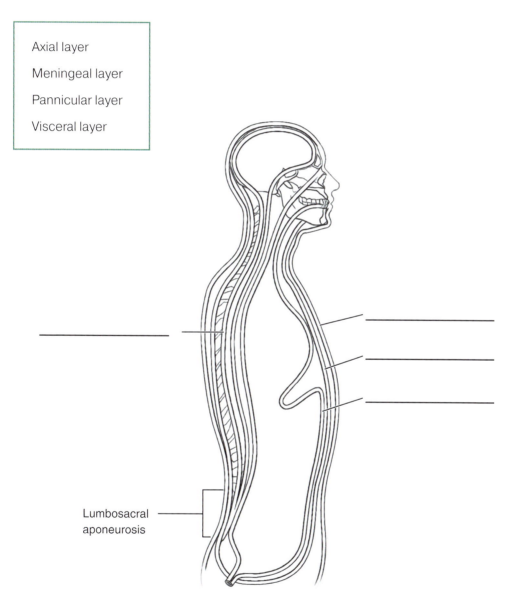

Lumbosacral aponeurosis

8: Neuromuscular and Myofascial Connections

Fascial Planes

Fascial planes are horizontal structural components of the deep fascia. These planes are thickened sheets of fascia inside body cavities that provide structural strength to the torso and support the major **2.** _____ _____

3. _____ and **4.** _____

Cranial base

Diaphragm

Pelvic floor

Thoracic inlet

Thoracic cavity

Abdominal cavity

Pelvic cavity

EXERCISE 7 • Mechanical Properties of Fascia

Historically, each mechanical property of fascia provided explanations and implications for the application of many manual therapy techniques. Complete the table below by defining each of the mechanical properties and describing the implications the physical property may have on the pace, pressure, duration, and/or movement utilized in manual therapy.

MECHANICAL PROPERTY	DEFINITION	IMPLICATION FOR PACE, PRESSURE, DURATION, AND/OR MOVEMENT
Viscoelasticity	1.	Decrease pace to allow for unwinding of tropocollagen; increased duration to allow complete unwinding; movement and pressure specific to technique and tissue being addressed
Thixotropy	2.	4.
Piezoelectricity	3.	5.

EXERCISE 8 • Fascial Receptors

Identify each statement below as characteristic of one of the four fascial mechanoreceptors. Use the following abbreviations to indicate your choices: Golgi organs (GO), Pacinian receptors (P), Ruffini's receptors (R), and interstitial myofascial receptors (IMF). If you need to refresh your memory, refer to Table 8.2 in your textbook.

_____ **1.** Located in spinal ligaments, as well as the epi-, peri-, and endomysium of muscle

_____ **2.** Specifically responsive to lateral and tangential stretch

_____ **3.** Stimulation causes decreased motor tone in related skeletal muscle

_____ **4.** Stimulation causes increased vagal activity that results in global relaxation and less emotional arousal

_____ **5.** Responsive to rapid pressure changes and vibrations

_____ **6.** Responsive to rapid and sustained pressure changes

_____ **7.** Only fascial mechanoreceptor found in the dura mater

_____ **8.** Input from these sensory receptors is key proprioceptive feedback for kinesthesia

_____ **9.** 50% of these mechanoreceptors are high threshold units and the other 50% are low threshold units

_____ **10.** Receptors at musculotendinous junction sense tension due to muscle contraction, while others in this category are only sensitive to strong stretch

EXERCISE 9 • Concepts in Posture, Balance, and Coordinated Movement

Match each term to its proper definition.

_____ **1.** Muscle tone

_____ **2.** Phasic muscle

_____ **3.** Muscle recruitment

_____ **4.** Motor tone

_____ **5.** Neurofascial loops

_____ **6.** Motor unit recruitment

_____ **7.** Fascial tone

_____ **8.** Postural muscle

A. Organizational pattern of stimulation and coactivation of muscle groups regulated by the cerebellum to produce complex coordinated movements

B. Skeletal muscle whose primary role is to create movement

C. Skeletal muscle that plays an essential role in maintaining the body's upright position

D. Low-grade tension created by smooth muscle cells within the fascia that is independent of motor tone in surrounding skeletal muscles; regulated by the ANS

E. Increasing the number of motor units stimulated to increase the force of a muscle; also known as graded response

F. A consistent state of low-grade tension generated through tonic contractions; palpated as firmness in the muscle

G. Natural firmness of a muscle created by its fluid and connective tissue elements

H. Reflexive neuronal pathways connecting the ANS to smooth muscle cells in the fascia

REVIEW QUIZ

Neuromuscular and Myofascial Connections

Multiple Choice: Select the one best answer.

1. What are the key mechanical properties of fascia?
   A. stretchable, adherent, and thixotropic
   B. excitable, extensible, and piezoelectricity
   C. tensegrity, viscoelasticity, and thixotropic
   D. viscoelasticity, piezoelectricity, and thixotropic

2. What is the best definition of muscle recruitment?
   A. the pattern of coactivation between muscle groups needed to create coordinated movement
   B. the sequential stimulation of muscle fascicles used to increase the strength of a contraction
   C. a pattern of stimulating agonist, synergist, and inhibiting antagonist needed to create smooth movement
   D. the sequential activation of all the muscle fibers needed to create a full muscle contration

3. Which of the neuromuscular reflex theories is the most effective at relieving a cramp?
   A. graded response
   B. all-or-none
   C. reciprocal inhibition
   D. sliding filament

4. What is the term for the process that increases the sensitivity of the muscle spindle?
   A. spindle hypersensitization
   B. gamma gain
   C. stretch reflex
   D. inverse stretch reflex

5. Which neuron loop of the muscle spindle stimulates skeletal muscle contraction?
   A. alpha
   B. beta
   C. gamma
   D. delta

6. All of the following manual therapy techniques except _____ employ some type of repositioning designed to reverse gamma gain and indirectly reduce muscle tension.
   A. positional release
   B. strain-counterstrain
   C. functional technique
   D. Rolfing

7. Which action provides the strongest stimulus to the GTOs and the inverse stretch reflex?
   A. sustained compression at the neuromuscular junctions
   B. bouncing types of stretch
   C. active muscle contraction
   D. slow gradual stretching

8. Gamma gain occurs in a muscle spindle when it is held in _____ for an extended time.
   A. a lengthened position
   B. eccentric contraction
   C. a shortened position
   D. tetanic contraction

9. In addition to being hypersensitive to moderate compression, other key characteristics of a trigger point include
   A. a common pattern of pain with pressure and a palpable nodule within a taut band of tissue.
   B. muscle sensitivity to full stretch and a palpable deficit in the muscle belly.
   C. a hard end feel that also recreates the pain complaint.
   D. palpation of the point, stretch, and an isometric resistive all recreate a predictable pattern of pain.

10. According to reciprocal inhibition, which muscle is inhibited when the biceps brachii is contracted?
    A. brachioradialis
    B. coracobrachialis
    C. deltoid
    D. triceps brachii

11. Which of these is believed to be a key element of the pathophysiology behind trigger point development?
    A. The presence of calcium outside of the sarcoplasmic reticulum causes actin and myosin bonding.
    B. A false stretch reflex report from the muscle spindle causes a local muscle contraction.
    C. There is compression being applied to the motor neuron causing the contraction.
    D. A fibrotic buildup within the sarcomeres maintains the actin-myosin bond.

12. The term used to describe the balance of tension and compression forces in the musculoskeletal system is
    A. thixotropic.
    B. viscoelastic.
    C. piezoelectric.
    D. tensegrity.

13. What is the functional relevance of the 11 horizontal fascial bands of the body?
    A. attach the appendages to the torso to help transmit core strength to movement
    B. provide some stability to the torso by strapping the soft anterior structures to the spine
    C. separate the abdominal from pelvic organs in the ventral cavity
    D. provide a medium for force transmission between body regions

14. What is the purpose of the four horizontal planes of fascia in the body?
    A. transmit force and compression from skeletal muscle contraction to all body regions
    B. serve as the primary spacers and tension strut between organs in the cavities
    C. provide broad and deeply invested attachments for thoracic and abdominal muscles
    D. structurally divide both anterior and posterior cavities and support blood vessels and nerves.

15. Which phrase best describes a tender point?
    A. contraction knot
    B. metabolic crisis
    C. always occurs in a taut band of myofascial tissue
    D. local spasm indicating a sensitized muscle spindle

16. According to Willard, the deepest of the four layers of fascia is the
    A. meningeal.
    B. visceral.
    C. pannicular.
    D. axial.

17. Which of Myers's myofascial trains connects the plantar fascia of the foot to the fascia on the forehead?
    A. spiral line
    B. deep back line
    C. superficial back line
    D. lateral line

18. The four horizontal facial planes include the diaphragm, cranial base, pelvic floor, and
    A. thoracic inlet.
    B. thoracolumbar aponeurosis.
    C. abdominal aponeurosis.
    D. linea alba.

19. Which mechanical property of fascia gives it the ability to extend and slowly rebound?
    A. viscoelasticity
    B. thixotropic
    C. piezoelectric
    D. stretchability

20. Which of the four types of fascial sensory receptors are particularly sensitive to lateral stretch, and stimulation of them leads to decreased sympathetic tone?
    A. Golgi organs
    B. Pacinian receptors
    C. Ruffini's receptors
    D. interstitial myofascial receptors

21. The most abundant type of fascial sensory receptor are the _____ receptors.
    A. Golgi
    B. Pacinian
    C. Ruffini's
    D. interstitial myofascial

22. Since 40%–45% of the neurons in a typical skeletal muscle nerve are sensory, and 80% of these are the interstitial myofascial receptors, it appears that the majority of sensory information provided by muscle and fascia is directed toward the
    A. coordination of movement.
    B. autonomic nervous system.
    C. maintenance of posture.
    D. regulation of muscle tone.

23. The presence of smooth muscle cells in fascia leads us to believe that manipulation of fascia may play an important role in the regulation of
    A. muscle tone.
    B. motor tone.
    C. heart rate.
    D. blood pressure.

24. The ability to sense movement is called
    A. proprioception.
    B. equilibrium.
    C. kinesthesia.
    D. movement awareness.

25. What type of skeletal muscle fiber is characterized as a red or slow-twitch fiber?
    A. phasic fibers
    B. collagen fibers
    C. Type II fibers
    D. Type I fibers

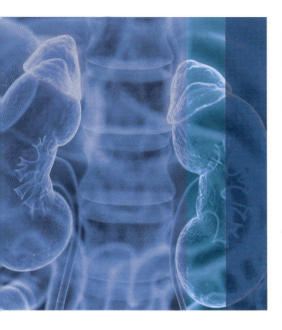

9

The Endocrine System

Use this list to choose learning exercises that will help you expand and solidify your understanding of key topics. To test your knowledge, try the Review Quiz at the end of the chapter.

Key Topics	Exercise
• System Terminology	1
• Components of the System and Their Location	2
• Comparing Endocrine and Nervous Communication	3
• Hormones: Classification and Methods of Action	4 & 5
• Endocrine Glands and Their Hormones	6 & 7
• Stress Responses	8

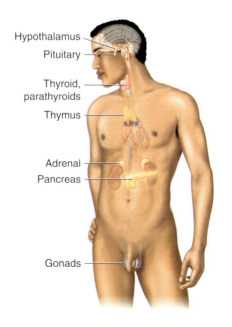

EXERCISE 1 • Endocrine System Crossword

Use this crossword to review and test your knowledge of the anatomy and physiology terms from Chapter 9.

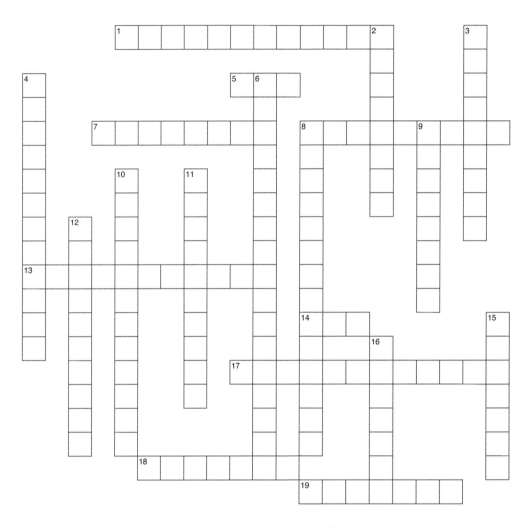

ACROSS

1. Another name for growth hormone.
5. Rate of oxygen consumption of the body at rest.
7. Steroid that acts as a male sex hormone.
8. Any hormone secreted by the adrenal cortex.
13. Effect created when two hormones work together to enhance or intensify the response of a target.
14. Also known as vasopressin.
17. These hormones do not require a second messenger to affect their target; includes steroid hormones.
18. A compound composed of a chain of 3–49 amino acids.
19. Synonym for suprarenal.

DOWN

2. Most hormone levels are regulated via this kind of feedback mechanism.
3. Master gland attached to the hypothalamus.
4. Effect created by a hormone working against another hormone.
6. Aldosterone is an example of this type of hormone released from the outer layer of the adrenal cortex.
8. Group of hormones that includes adrenaline and noradrenaline.
9. Important glucocorticoid with anti-inflammatory properties.
10. These hormones require a second messenger to affect their target.
11. This stage of the stress response includes longer-term endocrine activity; _____ reaction.
12. The pancreatic islets are also called the islets of _____.
15. Lipid-soluble hormone made from cholesterol.
16. Specialized chemical messenger released by an endocrine gland.

EXERCISE 2 • Locating Endocrine Glands

Color and identify each of the endocrine glands in the diagram below.

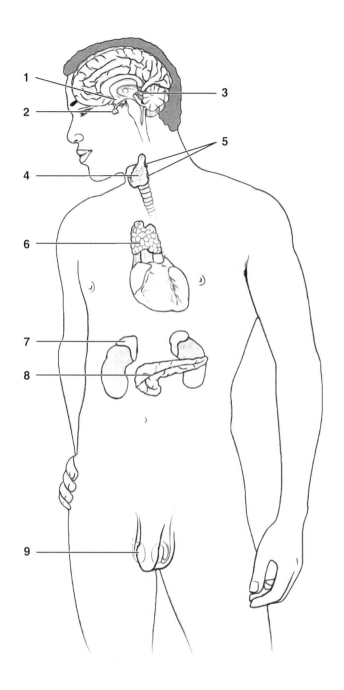

1. _____
2. _____
3. _____
4. _____
5. _____
6. _____
7. _____
8. _____
9. _____

EXERCISE 3 • Comparing the Communication Systems

Complete the table to compare and contrast important features and functions of the endocrine and nervous systems.

CHARACTERISTIC/FUNCTION	ENDOCRINE SYSTEM	NERVOUS SYSTEM
Primary organs of system connected and exclusive to the system (yes or no)	1.	2.
Speed of communication	3.	4.
Rate and type of physiologic changes controlled by the system	5.	6.
Anatomic connections between the systems	7.	8.
Method of signaling effector change	9.	10.

116   REVIEW GUIDE

EXERCISE 4 • Mechanisms of Hormone Action

There are two broad categories of hormones: water-soluble and lipid-soluble hormones. Completing the blanks as well as coloring and labeling the diagrams in this exercise will help you walk step by step through the two mechanisms of hormone action. You may want to do the fill-in exercise first and then color the diagrams, or vice versa. Since the answers for the fill-in exercise and the labels for the diagrams match, you may also choose to move back and forth between the two portions of the exercise. No matter how you choose to work, if you need to refresh your memory, refer to Figures 9.4 and 9.5 and the section on mechanisms of hormone action in your textbook.

1. _____ _____ hormones are recognized by receptors on the

2. _____ _____ , which bond with the hormone. This connection between

hormone and receptor activates a **3.** _____, which initiates the conversion of ATP in the

cytoplasm into **4.** _____. The presence of this substance activates proteins within the cell

that produce a designated **5.** _____ _____. This sequence of events is

called the **6.** _____ _____ _____ .

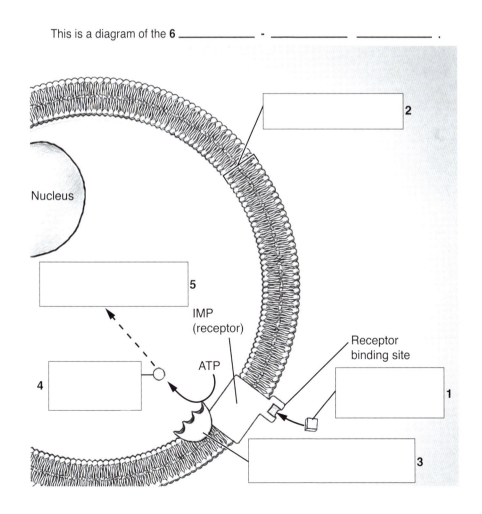

This is a diagram of the **6** _____ - _____ _____ .

9: The Endocrine System

In contrast, **7.** _____ _____ hormones are more direct because they are able to pass through the **8.** _____ _____ to bond with receptors in the **9.** _____. This forms a hormone-receptor complex that passes through the **10.** _____ _____ and activates a process in which specific genes (segments of **11.** _____) are copied onto an **12.** _____ molecule that then directs the production of a new **13.** _____ by the ribosomes. This substance alters the metabolic activity of the cell.

This is a diagram of direct mechanism used by **7.** _____ - _____ hormones.

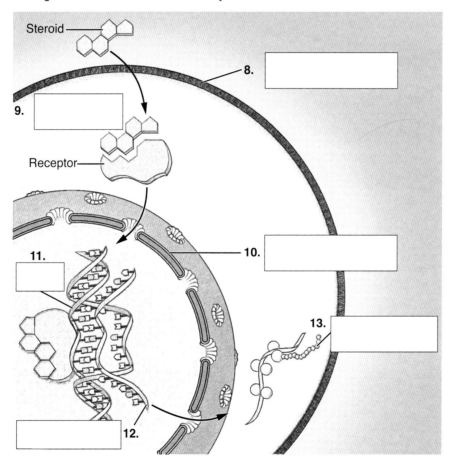

EXERCISE 5 • Stimulating and Regulating Hormone Activity

Most hormone levels and activity are regulated through negative feedback mechanisms. Color and label the diagram below to identify the components of the feedback loop. If you need to refresh your memory, refer to Figure 9.6 in your textbook.

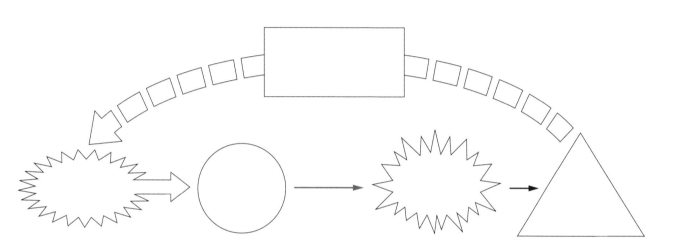

Endocrine gland
Physiologic response
Stimulus
Negative feedback
Hormone
Target cells or organ

List three types of stimuli that activate endocrine glands to release their hormones, and provide at least one example of each.

1. _____ ex. _____
2. _____ ex. _____
3. _____ ex. _____

EXERCISE 6 • Glands and Their Hormones

Complete the table by listing the hormones secreted for each endocrine gland identified in the diagram. The bullet points in the table & numbers in parentheses of the diagram let you know how many hormones you should be able to list.

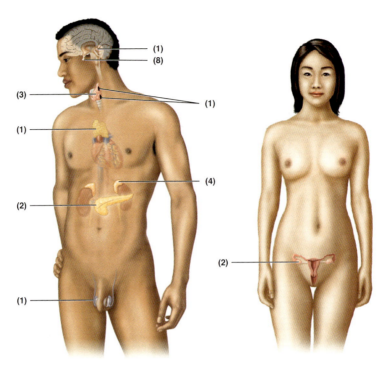

GLAND	HORMONES
Pineal	•
Anterior pituitary	• • • • • •
Posterior pituitary	• •
Thyroid	• • •
Parathyroids	•
Thymus	•
Adrenals	• • • •
Pancreas	• •
Ovaries	• •
Testes	•

120   REVIEW GUIDE

EXERCISE 7 • Matching Hormones and Physiologic Responses

Match each of these hormones with its physiologic effect.

_____ **1.** ACTH

_____ **2.** Glucagon

_____ **3.** PTH

_____ **4.** Testosterone

_____ **5.** Thymosin

_____ **6.** LH

_____ **7.** Cortisol

_____ **8.** GH

_____ **9.** Prolactin

_____ **10.** Adrenaline

_____ **11.** Oxytocin

_____ **12.** Estrogen

_____ **13.** Calcitonin

_____ **14.** Progesterone

_____ **15.** Thyroxine (T$_4$)

_____ **16.** Insulin

_____ **17.** Aldosterone

_____ **18.** Melatonin

A. Increases Na$^+$ retention, and thus water retention, to increase blood pressure; decreases K$^+$ in blood

B. Increases blood glucose and anti-inflammatory process, especially during stress response

C. Increases blood glucose; increases metabolism; prolongs body changes initiated by alarm response during stress

D. Maturation of ova; development and maintenance of secondary sex characteristics; prepares uterus for implantation

E. Development and maintenance of secondary sex characteristics; sperm production

F. Promotes growth of uterine lining and decreases uterine contractions to support pregnancy

G. Accelerates conversion of glycogen and other nutrients to glucose to increase glucose level in blood

H. Accelerates transport of glucose into cells to decrease glucose level in blood

I. Promotes maturation of T cells

J. Stimulates bone resorption to increase calcium level in blood, and production of calcitriol to increase Ca^{2+} absorption in digestive tract

K. Inhibits bone resorption and accelerates calcium uptake to decrease calcium level in blood

L. Increases metabolism

M. Triggers sleep

N. Stimulates uterine contraction and release of milk

O. Stimulates growth and increases metabolism

P. Stimulates milk production

Q. Increases secretion of hormones from testes and ovaries

R. Increases secretion of glucocorticoids from the adrenals

EXERCISE 8 • Diagramming Stress

Color and complete the flow chart below to outline the three stages of stress and the physiologic responses associated with each. If you need to refresh your memory, refer to Figure 9.16 in your textbook.

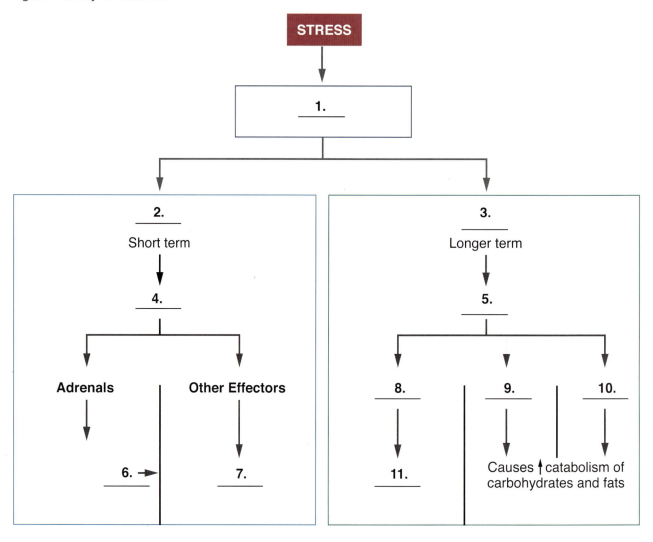

12. – occurs if the resistance response fails to combat the stress.

1. _____
2. _____
3. _____
4. _____
5. _____
6. _____

7. _____
8. _____
9. _____
10. _____
11. _____

12. _____

REVIEW QUIZ

The Endocrine System

Multiple Choice: Select the one best answer.

1. The four tropic hormones are thyroid-stimulating (TSH), adrenocorticotropic (ACTH), _____, and _____.
   A. somatotropin (SMT); gonadotropin (GT)
   B. antidiuretic (ADH); oxytocin (AT)
   C. follicle-stimulating (FSH); luteinizing (LH)
   D. vasopressin (VP); parathyroid-stimulating (PTS)

2. The functions of the endocrine system are body-wide communication and control of growth, development, and metabolism plus
   A. modulation of the stress response.
   B. stimulations of all visceral organ processes.
   C. regulation of heart and respiratory rates.
   D. homeostatic balance of the blood.

3. Which of the two chemical categories of hormones is the most prevalent in humans?
   A. steroidal
   B. lipid-soluble
   C. water-soluble
   D. semi-steroidal

4. The most prevalent method for hormones to stimulate action, and create a response, in their target organ is called the
   A. second-messenger mechanism.
   B. first-messenger theory.
   C. RAA pathway.
   D. nucleic-RNA cycle.

5. Which of these is a rare example of a hormone regulated via a positive feedback mechanism?
   A. insulin
   B. oxytocin
   C. thyroxine
   D. calcitonin

6. The two lobes of the pituitary are named for the different types of tissue and method of stimulation from the hypothalamus. The anterior lobe is the _____, and the posterior is called the _____.
   A. hypothesis; posteriohypothesis
   B. neurohypophysis; glandular-hypophysis
   C. adenohypophysis; neurohypophysis
   D. glandular-hypophysis; neurohypophysis

7. What structural characteristic distinguishes an endocrine gland from an exocrine gland?
   A. endocrine glands are attached to their target effector
   B. their small size and discreet locations
   C. they do not have a specific duct for their secretions
   D. their large number of sensory receptors

8. The three ways our body stimulates hormone release is via (1) changes in blood concentrations of a specific ion or nutrient, (2) hormonal stimulus from another endocrine gland, and (3)
   A. sympathetic chain stimulus.
   B. decreases in parasympathetic tone.
   C. neurologic stimulus of a specific gland.
   D. gastrointestinal pH changes.

9. In addition to the tropins, what other key hormone is released from the anterior pituitary?
   A. oxytocin
   B. ACTH
   C. releasing hormone
   D. growth hormone

10. Which hormone is released by the thyroid and increases cellular metabolism?
    A. thyroid-stimulating hormone
    B. thyrotropin
    C. calcitonin
    D. T_3 (triiodothyronine)

11. Where are the hormones oxytocin and antidiuretic produced?
    A. anterior pituitary
    B. posterior pituitary
    C. hypothalamus
    D. adrenals

12. Which hormone increases blood calcium levels by accelerating bone matrix breakdown?
    A. calcitonin
    B. parathyroid hormone
    C. growth hormone
    D. T_4

13. What is the name for the active form of vitamin D that accelerates absorption of calcium in the digestive tract?

   A. calcitriol
   B. parathyroid hormone
   C. charged D^3
   D. calcium-stimulating D

14. Which of the following is the target for ACTH?

   A. posterior pituitary
   B. kidneys
   C. adrenals
   D. adenohypophysis

15. What is the function of hormones secreted by the hypothalamus?

   A. stimulate or inhibit release of anterior pituitary hormones
   B. stimulate release of oxytocin
   C. inhibit the production of antidiuretic hormone
   D. regulate the autonomic nervous system

16. What is the function of aldosterone?

   A. increase urine production
   B. increase sodium retention
   C. decrease sodium retention
   D. decrease potassium secretion

17. What hormone is considered the primary glucocorticoid?

   A. glucagon
   B. insulin
   C. aldosterone
   D. cortisol

18. Which of the pancreatic islet cells produce insulin?

   A. alpha
   B. beta
   C. delta
   D. gamma

19. What is the function of insulin?

   A. increase blood glucose levels
   B. decrease glyconeogenesis
   C. decrease blood glucose levels
   D. increase glucose storage

20. Where is the hormone glucagon produced?

   A. adrenal cortex
   B. adrenal medulla
   C. posterior pituitary
   D. pancreas

21. The hormones that have the strongest effect on blood glucose levels include insulin, glucagon, glucocorticoids, and

   A. growth hormone.
   B. aldosterone.
   C. thymosin.
   D. parathyroid hormone.

22. When blood sodium levels are low, the adrenals secrete which hormone?

   A. cortisone
   B. aldosterone
   C. renin
   D. cortisol

23. Where is cortisol produced?

   A. adrenal medulla
   B. adrenal cortex
   C. pancreas
   D. adenohypophysis

24. What is the secondary effect of aldosterone?

   A. increased blood volume and blood pressure
   B. decreased blood pressure and pH
   C. support of inflammation and healing
   D. increased glycogenolysis

25. Which of the following would be considered a primary stress hormone?

   A. insulin
   B. oxytocin
   C. cortisol
   D. PTH

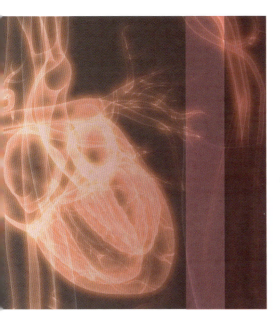

10

The Cardiovascular System

Use this list to choose learning exercises that will help you expand and solidify your understanding of key topics. To test your knowledge, try the Review Quiz at the end of the chapter.

Key Topics	Exercise
• System Terminology	1
• Blood Components	2
• Blood Vessels: Structure, Names, and Locations	3–6
• The Heart: Structure and Blood Flow	7–10
• The Cardiac Cycle	10
• Systemic Blood Flow and Circulation	11 & 12
• Blood Pressure Regulation	13
• Capillary Flow	14
• Stages of Tissue Healing	15

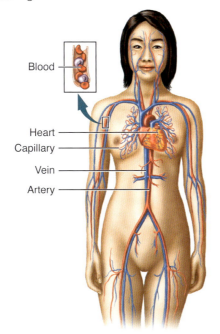

EXERCISE 1 • Cardiovascular Crossword

Use this crossword to review and test your knowledge of the general anatomy and physiology terms from Chapter 10.

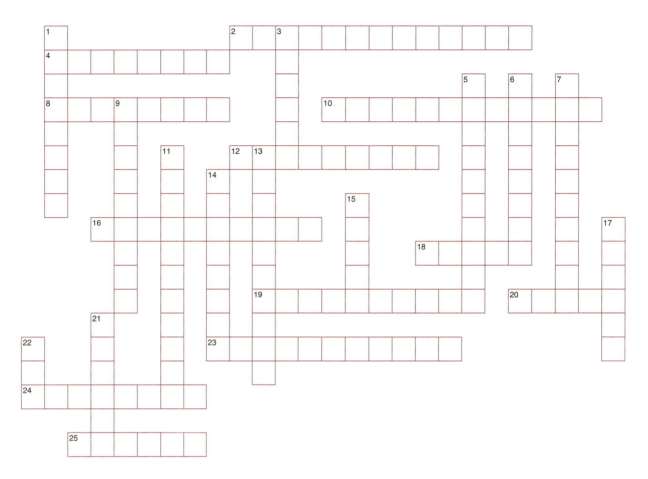

ACROSS

2. Blood cell production in the red bone marrow.
4. Local decrease in blood volume or flow.
8. Also called the proliferative stage of healing.
10. An organized network of _____ cardiac muscle cells creates the conduction system of the heart.
12. Reflexive contraction of muscles surrounding an injured area to help keep the area still and protected.
16. Starling forces produce a net _____ of fluids out of the capillaries.
18. In the pulmonary circuit, these blood vessels carry oxygen-rich blood.
19. A synonym for the visceral pericardium.
20. The palpable bulging of an artery in response to ventricular contraction that can be used to measure heart rate.
23. Process of blood clotting.
24. Also called a thrombocyte.
25. The fluid component of blood.

DOWN

1. Relaxation state in which the chambers of the heart dilate in order to fill with blood.
3. Valve located between the left atrium and ventricle.
5. The thick muscular layer of the heart.
6. A blood clot.
7. The _____ node is the pacemaker iof the heart.
9. A small artery.
11. An RBC.
13. Vessel elasticity, lumen size, and blood viscosity all contribute to _____ resistance within the cardiovascular network.
14. A bluish appearance of the skin, lips, or nail beds due to tissues not receiving enough oxygen.
15. Excess collection of fluid in the interstitial space.
17. A vessel that carries blood away from the heart.
21. Veins leaving the stomach, spleen, pancreas, and intestines merge to form this vein, which carries blood to the liver for cleansing.
22. Starling force produced by blood pressing out against the wall of a capillary.

126 REVIEW GUIDE

EXERCISE 2 • Matching Blood Components

Match the plasma components and formed elements below with the descriptions and characteristics offered.

_____ 1. Water

_____ 2. Hemoglobin

_____ 3. Erythrocytes

_____ 4. Thrombocytes

_____ 5. Globulins

_____ 6. Leukocytes

_____ 7. Albumins

_____ 8. Neutrophils

_____ 9. Fibrinogen

_____ 10. Lymphocytes

A. The most abundant type of protein found in plasma

B. Plasma proteins such as antibodies and complements

C. 90% of plasma is made up of this key component

D. Plasma protein that forms thin initial threads of a blood clot

E. Formed element present in the highest numbers in blood

F. Round cells with a prominent nucleus

G. Specialized agranular leukocytes

H. Formed elements essential for blood clotting

I. RBC protein that binds and carries O_2 and CO_2

J. Along with other granular leukocytes, this formed element plays a role in inflammation and tissue healing

EXERCISE 3 • Blood Vessel Structure

Place the name of the blood vessels shown within the numbered boxes of the diagram provided. Then, color and label the lettered items in the diagram to identify the layers of the vascular walls and other distinctive structural features of the blood vessels. If you need to refresh your memory, refer to Figure 10.3 in your textbook.

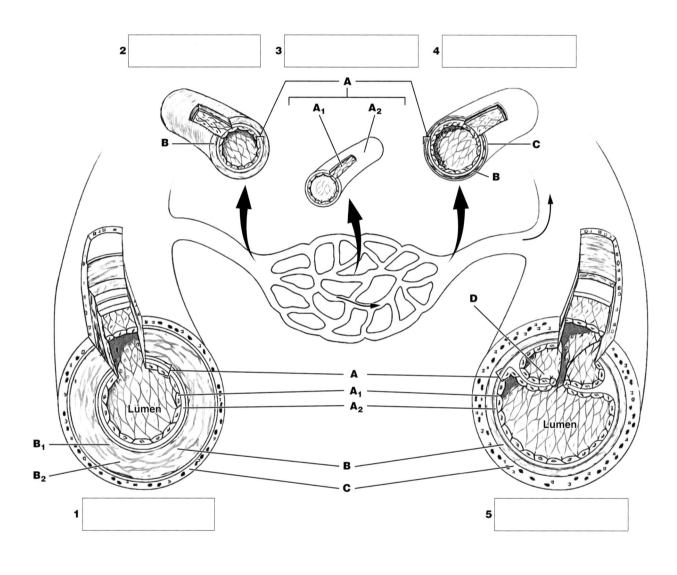

A _____

A₁ _____

A₂ _____

B _____

B₁ _____

B₂ _____

C _____

D _____

128   REVIEW GUIDE

EXERCISE 4 • Comparing and Contrasting Blood Vessels

Use the Venn diagram below to identify similarities and differences between arteries, capillaries, and veins. If you need to refresh your memory about structural characteristics and specific functions of the blood vessels, refer to Table 10.2 and the sections describing blood vessels in your textbook. To review instructions on how to use a Venn diagram, look at Chapter 6, Exercise 3, in this review guide. A characteristic common to all three types of vessels has been provided to help get you started.

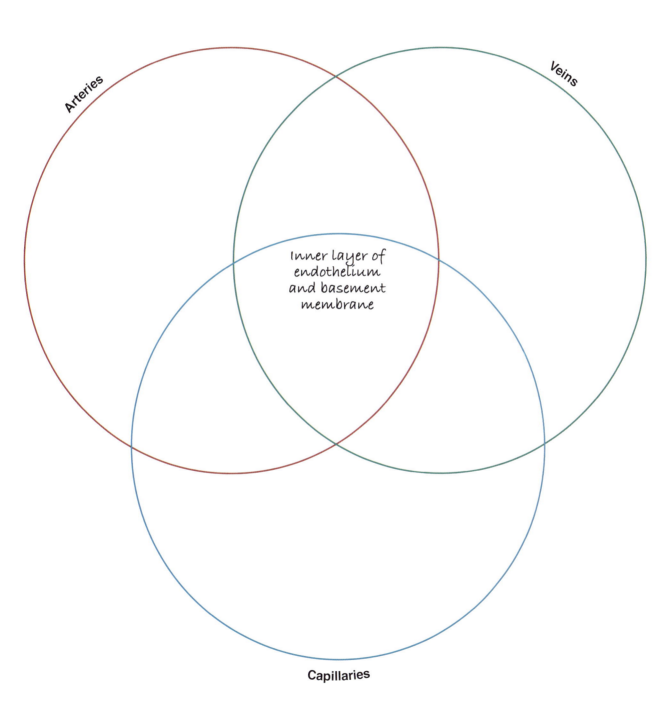

10: The Cardiovascular System

EXERCISE 5 • Primary Arteries of the Body

Match the artery with the letter identifying it on the diagram. Identify the common pulse points with a circle both on the diagram and in the list. Refer to Figure 10.4 in your textbook if you need to refresh your memory.

_____ 1. Temporal

_____ 2. Brachial

_____ 3. Dorsalis pedis

_____ 4. Common iliac

_____ 5. Radial

_____ 6. Femoral

_____ 7. Renal

_____ 8. Facial

_____ 9. Subclavian

_____ 10. Ulnar

_____ 11. Descending aorta

_____ 12. External carotid

_____ 13. Popliteal

_____ 14. Brachiocephalic trunk

_____ 15. Abdominal aorta

_____ 16. Common carotid

_____ 17. Axillary

_____ 18. Posterior tibial

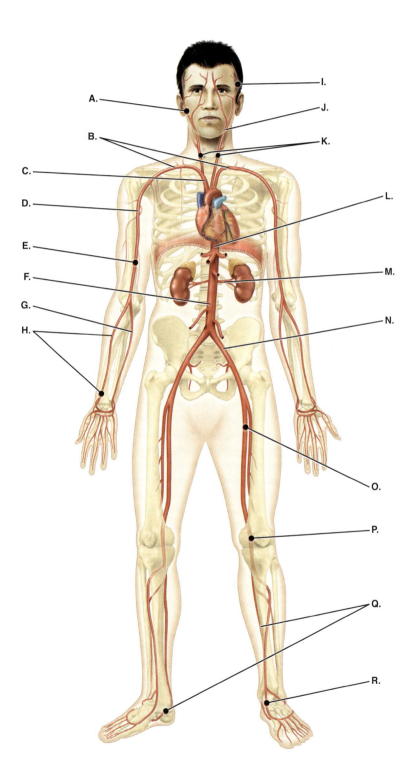

130 REVIEW GUIDE

EXERCISE 6 • Primary Veins of the Body

Match the vein with the letter identifying it on the diagram. If you need to refresh your memory refer to Figure 10.6 in your text.

_____ 1. Popliteal

_____ 2. Brachiocephalic

_____ 3. Superior vena cava

_____ 4. Inferior vena cava

_____ 5. Radial

_____ 6. Ulnar

_____ 7. Femoral

_____ 8. Internal iliac

_____ 9. Subclavian

_____ 10. Cephalic

_____ 11. Palmar arches

_____ 12. Digital

_____ 13. Brachial

_____ 14. Internal jugular

_____ 15. External jugular

_____ 16. Axillary

_____ 17. Median cubital

_____ 18. Basilic

_____ 19. Saphenous

_____ 20. Dorsal venous arch

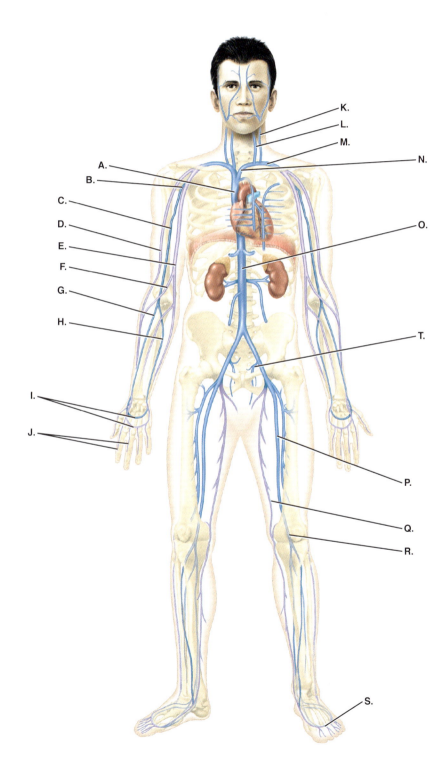

10: The Cardiovascular System   131

EXERCISE 7 • The Layers of the Heart

Using the diagram provided, color and label the layers of the heart wall and the sack surrounding the heart. Bracket the layers that actually form the heart wall. If you need to refresh your memory, refer to Figure 10.7 in your textbook.

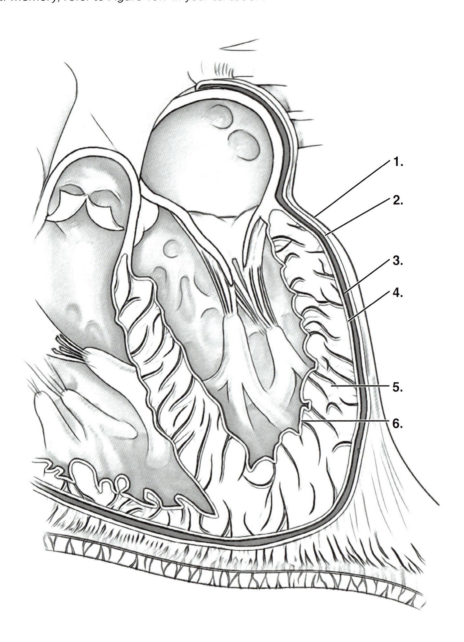

1. _____
2. _____
3. _____
4. _____
5. _____
6. _____

EXERCISE 8 • Blood Flow through the Heart

Color and label the great vessels and structures of the heart identified in the diagram below. If you need to refresh your memory, refer to Figure 10.8 in your textbook.

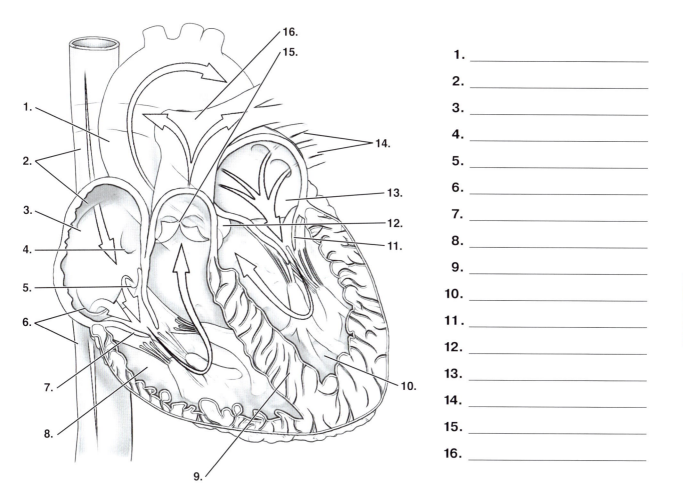

1. _____
2. _____
3. _____
4. _____
5. _____
6. _____
7. _____
8. _____
9. _____
10. _____
11. _____
12. _____
13. _____
14. _____
15. _____
16. _____

Beginning with the right atrium (#1), number the following list to designate the order a blood cell would circulate through each structure.

__1__ Right atrium
_____ Left atrium
_____ Right ventricle
_____ Left ventricle
_____ Bicuspid valve
_____ Tricuspid valve
_____ Aortic valve

_____ Pulmonary valve
_____ Aorta
_____ Vena cavae
_____ Pulmonary veins
_____ Pulmonary arteries
_____ Systemic capillaries
_____ Lung capillaries

10: The Cardiovascular System   133

EXERCISE 9 • The Conduction System of the Heart

Complete the matching exercise to identify the components of the heart's conduction system.

_____ **1.** Atrioventricular node

_____ **2.** Purkinje fibers

_____ **3.** AV bundle

_____ **4.** Bundle branches

_____ **5.** Sinoatrial node

A. Pacemaker; initiates signal

B. Carries signal to the intraventricular septum

C. Convey signal to apex of the heart

D. Delays signal to allow contraction of atria

E. Carry signal up through the ventricles

Explain the numbered steps on the diagram to outline the path a signal passes across the heart to coordinate contraction. If you need to refresh your memory, refer to Figure 10.10B in your textbook.

1. _____

_____

_____

_____

2. _____

_____

_____

_____

3. _____

_____

_____

_____

4. _____

_____

_____

_____

_____

5. _____

_____

_____

_____

6. _____

_____

_____

_____

_____

134   REVIEW GUIDE

EXERCISE 10 • The Cardiac Cycle

Complete the description of each stage of the cardiac cycle by circling the contraction state of the atria and ventricles, circling the position of the valves, and describing the flow of blood.

Relaxation Phase

Atria are relaxed or contracted

Ventricles are relaxed or contracted

Semilunar valves are open or closed

AV valves are open or closed

Blood flows from _____ to _____

Atrial Systole

Atria are relaxed or contracted

Ventricles are relaxed or contracted

Semilunar valves are open or closed

AV valves are open or closed

Blood flows from _____ to _____

Ventricular Systole

Atria are relaxed or contracted

Ventricles are relaxed or contracted

Semilunar valves are open or closed

AV valves are open or closed

Blood flows from _____ to _____

EXERCISE 11 • Cardiovascular Circulation

Color and label the schematic representation of cardiovascular circulation. Use the list of terms provided for your labels. Notice that the right and left sides of the heart are already designated. Color blood vessels that carry oxygenated blood red while making vessels that carry deoxygenated blood blue. Color sites of gas exchange half and half. If you need to refresh your memory, refer to Figures 10.8B and 10.12 in your textbook.

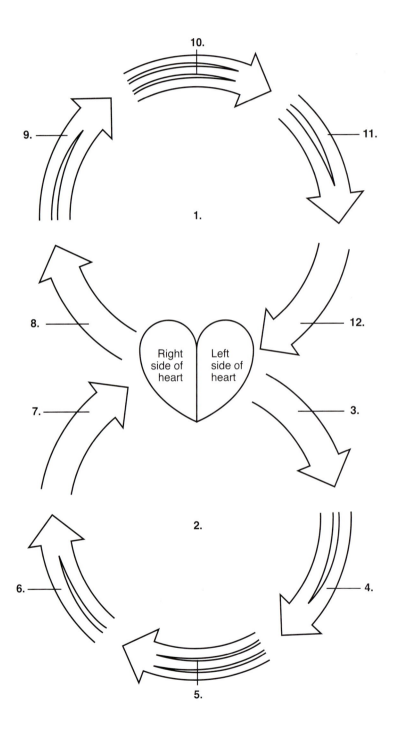

Pulmonary circuit
Systemic circuit
Aorta
Pulmonary arteries
Pulmonary arterioles
Pulmonary capillaries
Pulmonary veins
Pulmonary venules
Superior and inferior vena cavae
Systemic arterioles
Systemic capillaries
Systemic venules

1. _____
2. _____
3. _____
4. _____
5. _____
6. _____
7. _____
8. _____
9. _____
10. _____

EXERCISE 12 • Blood Flow

Blood moves through the different vessels of the cardiovascular network through a variety of forces.

Arterial blood flow is driven by the combined forces of **1.** _____

_____ and **2.** _____ _____.

Blood flow into the capillaries is controlled by the precapillary sphincters that constrict and dilate to control

both the **3.** _____ and the **4.** _____ of flow into the capillaries.

Venous flow is driven by **5.** _____ _____ _____

that apply external compression to the veins. One-way **6.** _____ assist venous flow by

creating shorter segments for blood to travel. In the ventral cavities the driving force for venous flow is the

7. _____ _____.

EXERCISE 13 • Blood Pressure Regulation

Blood pressure is a measurement of the **1.** _____

_____. This measurement consists of two numbers, stated

in terms of millimeters of mercury (mm Hg). The higher number is the **2.** _____ pressure,

which represents the pressure generated during **3.** _____ _____.

The **4.** _____ pressure is a lower number that represents the pressure in the arteries

when the **5.** _____ _____.

Blood pressure changes occur throughout the day to meet circulatory demands.
Mark each example listed below with either a ⬆ to indicate a factor that would increase blood pressure or a ⬇
to indicate a factor that would decrease blood pressure.

_____ **6.** Increased viscosity of the blood

_____ **7.** Hardening of the arteries

_____ **8.** Relaxation

_____ **9.** Physical exertion

_____ **10.** Use of medications to thin the blood

_____ **11.** Aldosterone release from the adrenals

_____ **12.** Increased elasticity of the vascular wall

EXERCISE 14 • Capillary Flow

Capillary exchange between blood and the interstitium involves the movement of particles or solutes, as well as fluids. Solutes move through the wall of the capillary via **1.** _____ and include substances such as **2.** _____, _____, and

_____ _____.

Fluid is exchanged through a combination of two hydrostatic and two osmotic pressures collectively referred to as **3.** _____ _____. The two hydrostatic pressures are

• **4.** _____ _____ pressure, or CFP, created by blood inside the capillary pushing outward against its wall.

• **5.** _____ _____ pressure, or IFP, created by interstitial fluid pressing inward against the capillary wall.

The two osmotic pressures are

• **6.** _____ _____ pressure, or POP, the osmotic pressure created by the **7.** _____ content of the blood inside the capillary.

• **8.** _____ _____ pressure, or IOP, an osmotic pressure created by the protein content of interstitial fluid.

The movement of plasma and its dissolved solutes out of the blood and into the interstitium is called

9. _____, while **10.** _____ refers to the movement of substances back into the capillary bed. Both **11.** _____ and IOP create filtration, whereas

12. _____ and POP are the forces involved in reabsorption. In healthy tissue, the dominant Starling force throughout the capillary bed is CFP, causing **13.** _____ to occur along the capillary.

EXERCISE 15 • Stages of Tissue Healing

Complete the table by filling in the key physiologic events that occur during each stage of the tissue healing process.

STAGE OF HEALING	KEY PHYSIOLOGIC EVENTS
ACUTE OR 1._____ **STAGE**	**2.** • Hemorrhage and _____ • Muscle spasm and _____ • _____ • _____
SUBACUTE OR 3._____ **STAGE**	**4.** • Increased numbers of _____ • Decreased numbers of _____ • Healing begins with _____
MATURATION STAGE	**5.** • Collagen remodeling based on _____

REVIEW QUIZ

The Cardiovascular System

Multiple Choice: Select the one best answer.

1. In addition to transporting nutrients and wastes, and playing a major role in the body's immune responses, the cardiovascular system also helps regulate
   - A. lymphatic flow, cardiac volume, and rate of healing.
   - B. core temperature, tissue health, and blood pressure.
   - C. body temperature, pH, and fluid balance.
   - D. rate of healing, blood pressure, and circadian rhythm.

2. What is the correct anatomic term for a red blood cell?
   - A. leukocyte
   - B. thrombocyte
   - C. erythrocyte
   - D. fibrocyte

3. Which formed elements play the largest role in immune responses?
   - A. leukocytes
   - B. erythrocytes
   - C. plasma
   - D. thrombocytes

4. What is the primary component of plasma?
   - A. albumin
   - B. platelets
   - C. fibrinogen
   - D. water

5. What is the other term for platelets?
   - A. fibrocytes
   - B. thrombocytes
   - C. leukocytes
   - D. lymphocytes

6. What is the term for the three-stage physiologic process that stops bleeding or blood flow?
   - A. thrombosis
   - B. cardio-stenosis
   - C. coagulation
   - D. hemostasis

7. What are the two major divisions or circuits of the cardiovascular system?
   - A. arterial and venous
   - B. pulmonary and systemic
   - C. internal and external systemic
   - D. muscular and visceral

8. Why is the muscular layer in arteries thicker than that in veins?
   - A. Arteries must contract to propel blood forward and veins don't need to.
   - B. It makes them more resilient and creates a recoil that is important for arterial flow.
   - C. It helps protect arteries from trauma.
   - D. The thinner muscle in veins can contract more rapidly than the thicker layer in arteries.

9. What smooth muscle ring of tissue in blood vessels regulates the volume and rate of blood flow into the capillaries?
   - A. post-arteriole gate
   - B. prevenule sphincter
   - C. capillary endothelium
   - D. precapillary sphincter

10. Which major artery delivers blood to the upper extremities?
    - A. carotid
    - B. brachial
    - C. subclavian
    - D. descending aorta

11. Where is the saphenous vein located?
    - A. middle of the cubital fossa
    - B. the abdominopelvic cavity
    - C. along the lateral aspect of the upper extremity
    - D. along the medial aspect of the lower extremity

12. Which of these blood vessels carries deoxygenated blood into the liver?
    - A. portal vein
    - B. hepatic vein
    - C. splenic vein
    - D. inferior mesenteric

13. The baroreceptors that sense blood pressure are located in which major blood vessel?
    - A. carotid artery
    - B. abdominal aorta
    - C. jugular vein
    - D. pulmonary artery

14. What is the function of the pericardium?
    A. provides nutrient-waste exchange for the heart
    B. applies an external compression to the heart that strengthens the contractions
    C. firmly anchors the heart to the primary vessels
    D. acts as a protective covering that secretes serous fluid to decrease friction over the heart as it contracts

15. Which blood vessel carries blood from the heart to the lungs?
    A. pulmonary vein
    B. pulmonary artery
    C. respiratory aorta
    D. thoracic artery

16. What is the name of the heart valve located between the right atrium and ventricle?
    A. mitral
    B. bicuspid
    C. tricuspid
    D. pulmonary

17. Which chamber of the heart pumps blood into the systemic circuit of circulation?
    A. left ventrical
    B. right ventrical
    C. left atrium
    D. right atrium

18. Which chamber of the heart receives blood from the inferior vena cava?
    A. left ventrical
    B. right ventrical
    C. left atrium
    D. right atrium

19. Which of the Starling forces is the dominant force behind capillary filtration?
    A. interstitial fluid pressure
    B. capillary fluid pressure
    C. plasma oncotic pressure
    D. interstitial oncotic pressure

20. The amount of pressure exerted by blood against the walls of the arteries is called
    A. peripheral resistance.
    B. arterial pressure.
    C. blood pressure.
    D. essential pressure.

21. Which portion of the cardiac conduction system serves as the pacemaker?
    A. left bundle branch
    B. sinoatrial node
    C. AV node
    D. Purkinje fibers

22. The primary influences over venous flow are the one-way valves and
    A. skeletal muscle contraction.
    B. ventricular systole.
    C. the pulse.
    D. myocardial recoil.

23. In what stage of tissue healing do we see margination and hematoma organization?
    A. acute
    B. subacute
    C. chronic
    D. maturation mobility

24. What action could be considered the safest and most important for manual therapists to do during the healing cycle to assure proper repair, tissue alignment, strength, and pliability?
    A. Introduce direct cross-fiber friction in the acute stage.
    B. Begin alternating heat and cold applications in the subacute phase.
    C. Avoid any direct tissue manipulation until maturation stage.
    D. Encourage pain-free movement throughout all stages.

25. What is the main cause of secondary edema after acute sprains and strains?
    A. muscle splinting
    B. granulation tissue formation
    C. fibrocyte migration
    D. increased interstitial oncotic pressure

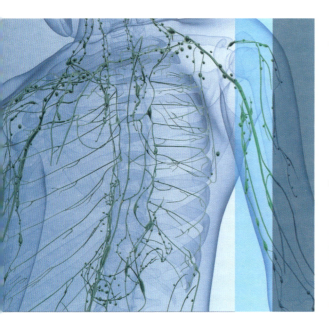

11

The Lymphatic System

Use this list to choose learning exercises that will help you expand and solidify your understanding of key topics. To test your knowledge, try the Review Quiz at the end of the chapter.

Key Topics	Exercise
• System Terminology	1
• Lymph Vessels and Nodes: Network and Functions	2–4
• Edema Uptake and Lymph Flow	5, 6, 8
• Catchments and Watersheds	7
• Types of Edema	9

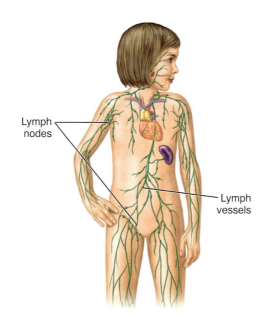

EXERCISE 1 • Lymphatic System Crossword

Use this crossword to review and test your knowledge of some of the lymphatic system's structures and functions.

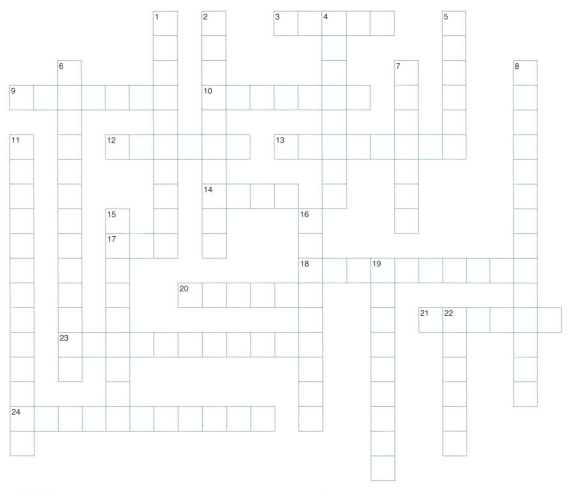

ACROSS

3. The primary component of lymph.
9. The first capillaries in the lymphatic network are _____ vessels.
10. Lymphedema due to a congenital defect in the lymphatic system is classified as _____ lymphedema.
12. The epithelial cells of initial vessels overlap and have this type of filament attached.
13. Specialized lymph capillaries that absorb fat from the small intestine.
14. In contrast to the cardiovascular system, the lymphatic system is _____, because it is a one-way system, not a circuit.
17. It regulates the contractile rate of collectors.
18. These projections divide the interior space of a lymph node into sinuses.
20. When interstitial fluid is drawn into the lymphatic vessels.
21. A segment of a collector.
23. Specialized WBCs found in high concentrations in lymph.
24. An end-to-end arrangement of lymph vessels found at watersheds.

DOWN

1. The primary lymphatic vessels; lymphangia.
2. A specific lymphatic drainage region.
4. This duct collects lymph from the upper left and both lower quadrants of the body.
5. Initial vessels are separated from pre-collectors with one-way _____.
6. Collecting well at the base of the thoracic duct.
7. Type of edema related to cardiovascular dysfunction.
8. This junction is also called the lymphatic terminus.
11. Fluid outside the cell is called _____ fluid.
15. Another name for a lymph node bed.
16. The zone between two lymphotomes.
19. Deep _____ and skeletal muscle contraction are both external influences on lymphatic flow.
22. An island of lymphocytes located within a sinus of a lymph node.

EXERCISE 2 • The Lymphatic Vessels

Complete the table, filling in key structural and functional information about the vessels of the lymphatic network. Notice that the table is organized from the smallest to the largest vessels.

LYMPHATIC VESSELS	LOCATION & STRUCTURE	FUNCTION
1. Capillaries or _____ _____	**2.** Located in _____ • Snub-nosed or _____attached • Has _____ _____attached to epithelial cells to help pull the capillary open	Entry point for fluid uptake in lymph vessel network
Pre-collectors	**3.** Located in superficial _____ • Wall is several layers of _____ cells • A single _____ _____ at the junction between it and the primary vessel	**4.** Collect lymph from several _____ _____
5. The primary vessels or _____	**6.** Superficial vessels located in dermis; deeper vessels are _____ or in deep fascia. • Divided into segments called _____ by one-way valves • Have spiral _____ within their walls	**7.** Collect lymph from several _____, and carry it into a specific lymph node bed
8. Larger primary vessels called _____ **carry lymph toward the deep ducts.**	**9.** Located deep and alongside major _____ • Intralymphatic valves are spaced _____ _____ than in the collectors.	**10.** Carry lymph out of the lymph node bed or _____
Lymphatic ducts	**11.** Located deep within tissue of right quadrant and _____ cavities • The _____ _____ is an enlarged collecting well at the base of the _____ _____.	**12.** Right lymphatic duct collects all lymph from upper right quadrant and returns it to right _____ vein. Thoracic duct collects lymph from three-quarters of the body, including upper left quadrant and _____ _____ quadrants, then returns it to the left subclavian vein.

EXERCISE 3 • Structure and Function of a Lymph Node

Lymph nodes are small specialized **1.** _____ _____ interspersed along the length of the **2.** _____. They are scattered along the lymphatic pathway and also found in clusters called **3.** _____ _____ _____ or **4.** _____. Lymph nodes function as **5.** _____, removing particulate matter such as **6.** _____ _____, along with **7.** _____ from lymph as it passes through. Additionally, lymph nodes contain numerous specialized lymph cells called **8.** _____, making the nodes primary sites for specific immune responses.

Label the diagram to review the structure of a lymph node. If you need to refresh your memory, refer to Figure 11.11A in your textbook.

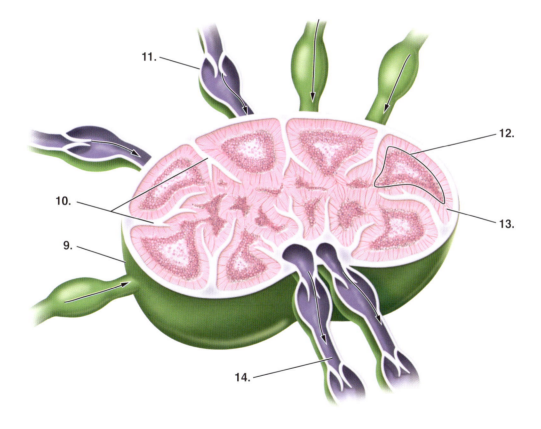

9. _____
10. _____
11. _____

12. _____
13. _____
14. _____

11: The Lymphatic System

EXERCISE 4 • The Lymphatic Network

Use the letters associated with the structures listed in the box to label the diagram.
If you need to refresh your memory, refer to Figure 11.2 in the textbook.

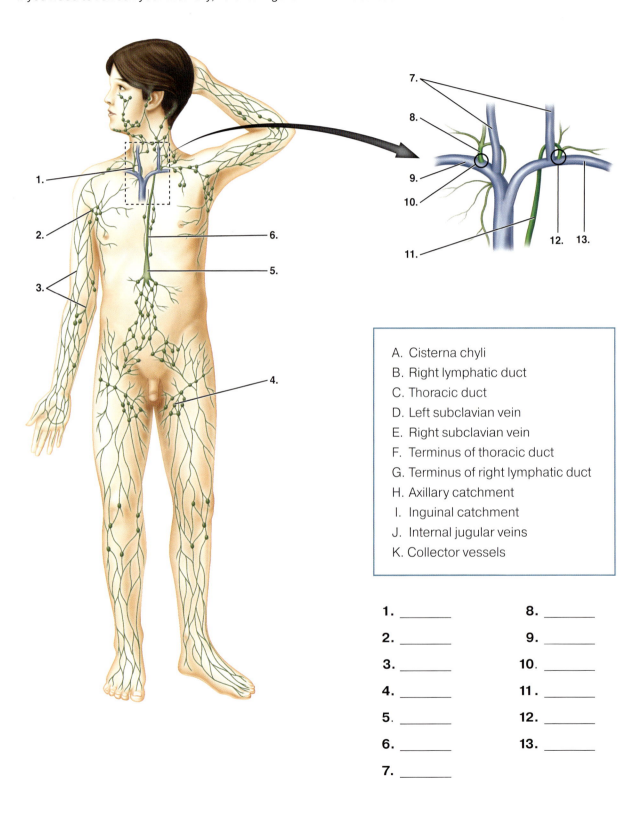

A. Cisterna chyli
B. Right lymphatic duct
C. Thoracic duct
D. Left subclavian vein
E. Right subclavian vein
F. Terminus of thoracic duct
G. Terminus of right lymphatic duct
H. Axillary catchment
I. Inguinal catchment
J. Internal jugular veins
K. Collector vessels

1. _____   8. _____
2. _____   9. _____
3. _____   10. _____
4. _____   11. _____
5. _____   12. _____
6. _____   13. _____
7. _____

146 REVIEW GUIDE

EXERCISE 5 • Edema Uptake Versus Lymphatic Flow

While interdependent, the processes of edema uptake and lymphatic flow are two different processes each facilitated by different structural characteristics and physiologic mechanisms.

Mark each of these physiologic processes or structural features as either EU to indicate it is a primary influence on edema uptake or LF if more related to lymph flow.

_____ **1.** Autonomic nervous system stimulation of smooth muscle contraction within the lymphangia

_____ **2.** Manually moving superficial fluid across a watershed to less congested lymphotomes

_____ **3.** External manipulation of tissue that applies a light stretch and release of the epidermis

_____ **4.** When interstitial fluid volumes increase, anchor filaments pull epithelial flaps of initial vessels open

_____ **5.** Anastomoses

_____ **6.** Negative pressure inside the lymphatic system

_____ **7.** No valves in initial vessels

_____ **8.** One-way valves inside the collector vessels

_____ **9.** Edema creates increased hydrostatic pressure in the interstitium

EXERCISE 6 • Mechanisms of Lymph Flow

Complete the concept map to identify the physiologic mechanisms that create and support lymph flow.

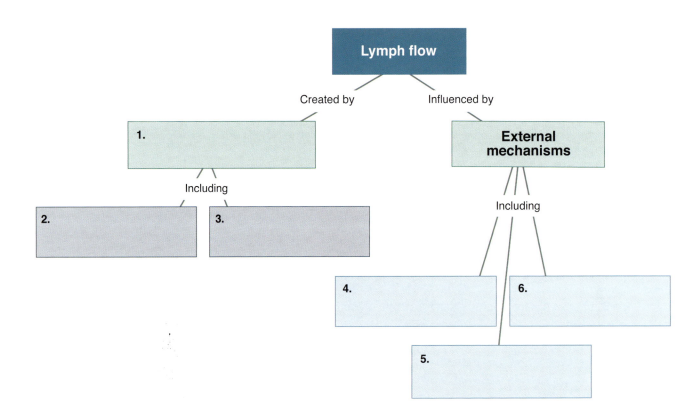

EXERCISE 7 • Catchments and Watersheds

Draw in the missing major watershed lines, and add dots to indicate the location of the major catchments. Then draw one or two arrows to indicate lymph flow within each area. To refresh your memory or check your work, refer to Figures 11.12 and 11.14 in the textbook.

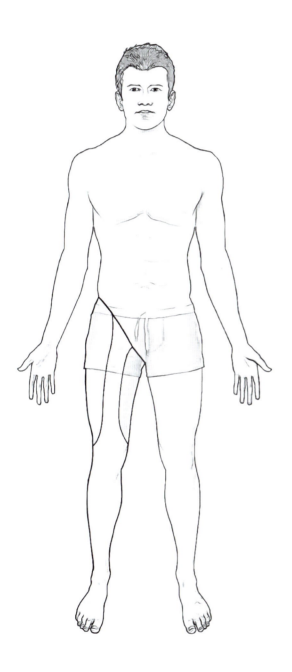
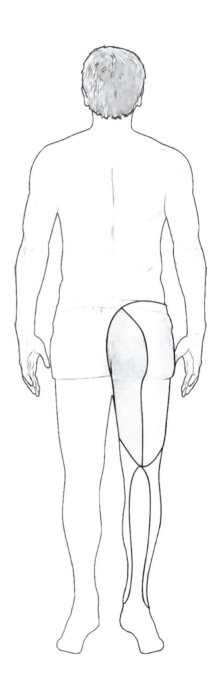

EXERCISE 8 • Routes of Lymph Flow

Use the list of lymphatic structures to outline routes of lymphatic flow. Beginning with edema uptake in the specific regions identified, place the letter of the structures into their proper sequence. Note that some structures may be a part of multiple routes.

A. Thoracic duct	G. Popliteal catchment
B. Right lymphatic duct	H. Anterior thigh lymphotomes
C. Terminus	I. Anterior leg lymphotomes
D. Axillary catchment	J. Posterior leg lymphotomes
E. Inguinal catchment	K. Medial arm lymphotomes
F. Cisterna chyli	L. Lateral arm lymphotomes

Edema Uptake   **Natural Flow Pattern**

@ anterior thigh   → 1. ____   → 2. ____   → 3. ____   → 4. ____   → 5. ____

@ right medial wrist   → 1. ____   → 2. ____   → 3. ____   → 4. ____

@ calf   → 1. ____   → 2. ____   → 3. ____   → 4. ____   → 5. ____   → 6. ____

@ right rib cage   → 1. ____   → 2. ____   → 3. ____

@ left lateral elbow   → 1. ____   → 2. ____   → 3. ____

@ anterior ankle   → 1. ____   → 2. ____   → 3. ____   → 4. ____   → 5. ____   → 6. ____

EXERCISE 9 • Types of Edema

Complete the table that compares and contrasts the different types of edema.

TYPE OF EDEMA	DEFINITION	EXAMPLES/ETIOLOGY
PRIMARY LYMPHEDEMA	1.	2.
3.	Edema due to damage to lymphatic system	4. Surgery, as well as . . . • •
5.	6.	7. Hypertension, obesity, as well as . . . • •
TRAUMATIC EDEMA	8.	9.

11: The Lymphatic System   151

REVIEW QUIZ

The Lymphatic System

Multiple Choice: Select the one best answer.

1. What are the functions of the lymphatic system?
   A. absorb fats from the digestive tract, return fluids and proteins to blood, and carry out several primary immune responses
   B. cleanse the interstitial fluid, facilitate venous flow, and initiate tissue healing
   C. play a key role in developing immunity, manage edema, and facilitate capillary exchange
   D. absorb vitamin D from the intestines, carry out immune responses, and manage edema

2. Where are the initial capillaries of the lymphatic system located?
   A. in the dermal layer of skin
   B. alongside the major arteries of the ventral cavities
   C. entwined in the interstitial spaces of the cardiovascular capillaries
   D. just superficial to all major veins

3. In addition to water and electrolytes, what are the other primary components of lymph?
   A. proteins, carbohydrates, lipids, and vitamins
   B. lymphocytes and neutrophils, proteins, nitrogen, and carbon dioxide
   C. foreign substances, hormones, metabolic waste, and macrophages
   D. cells, proteins, foreign substances, and long-chain fatty acids

4. What is the function of the pre-collector vessels?
   A. interstitial fluid uptake
   B. carry lymph into the catchments
   C. provide a channel through the epidermis to collector vessels
   D. gather fluid from multiple initial capillaries and transport to the collectors

5. Which of these statements is the best definition of anastomosis?
   A. the smallest functional unit of the collecting vessels
   B. a group of pre-collectors that connect different collectors for lymph transfer
   C. a group of larger collectors that carry lymph out of the catchments
   D. the area in subepidermis where the majority of the pre-collectors are located

6. Since the epidermis does not contain blood or lymph vessels, how does interstitial fluid from the skin get into the network of lymphatic vessels?
   A. specialized epithelial pores in the superficial layer of dermis
   B. the microscopic tubular network of the cytoskeleton in the epidermis
   C. nonstructural pathways between cells called pre-lymphatic channels
   D. the intercellular fluid pathway made up of lymphocytes

7. What is the purpose of the one-way valves in veins and collecting vessels of the lymphatic system?
   A. increase the force of propulsion of fluid through the vessels
   B. prevent backflow of fluid and divide the vessels into smaller segments
   C. provide extra surface area in the vessel for nutrient and waste exchange
   D. create extra resistance to fluid flow to mediate blood pressure

8. What is the name of the lymphovenous junction where fluid is returned to the cardiovascular system?
   A. lymphatic jugular junction
   B. cardio-lymphatic junction
   C. cisterna chyli
   D. terminus

9. What are the two primary watersheds on both the anterior and posterior torso?
   A. anterior clavicular and posterior umbilical
   B. diaphragmatic and sagittal
   C. supraclavicular and popliteal
   D. sagittal and umbilical

10. How much of the fluid filtered out of cardiovascular capillaries must be absorbed into the lymphatic capillaries?
    A. 100%
    B. 50%
    C. 0%
    D. 10%

152   REVIEW GUIDE

11. In order for edema or fluid uptake to occur, the flap cells of the initial vessels must be pulled open, and

   A. the individual's blood pressure must be within the normal range.
   B. there must be negative pressure inside the lymphatic vessel network.
   C. there must be positive pressure inside the lymphatic vessels.
   D. the rate of lymphangion contractions must be no higher than 6.

12. Which of the following statements best describes the function of the cisterna chyli?

   A. serves as the largest lymph node bed in the body
   B. collecting well for lymph at the base of the thoracic duct
   C. heart of the lymphatic system that pumps lymph through the entire system
   D. junction where lymph is returned to the cardiovascular system

13. One-way valves are important structural features in several lymph vessels, but are not found in

   A. collecting vessels.
   B. lymphatic trunks.
   C. initial capillaries.
   D. right lymphatic duct.

14. In addition to gravity, what other external forces provide key stimulus to lymph flow?

   A. increased arterial flow and properly hydrated tissue
   B. respiratory pump and skeletal muscle contraction
   C. the sodium and calcium pumps in muscles
   D. decreased arterial flow and abdominal breathing

15. A group of lymphatic vessels that drain lymph from a specific region of the body into a specific catchment are called

   A. collecting vessels.
   B. angions.
   C. deep trunks.
   D. lymphotomes.

16. What catchment receives lymph from the anterior leg and all regions of the thigh?

   A. inguinal
   B. popliteal
   C. perineal
   D. patellar

17. Which of the following are considered the two primary internal forces for creating and maintaining lymph flow?

   A. respiratory and skeletal muscle pumps
   B. arterial pulse and angion contraction
   C. siphon effect and autonomic angion contraction
   D. soft tissue stretch and release

18. Arterial flow and pulse have a major influence on lymph flow through which portion of the lymph system?

   A. anastomosis
   B. lymphatic trunks
   C. pre-collectors
   D. catchments

19. Swelling related to hypertension and obesity is called

   A. primary lymphedema.
   B. traumatic edema.
   C. secondary lymphedema.
   D. dynamic edema.

20. A dysfunction in the lymphatic system that results in swelling of an entire body area is called

   A. edema.
   B. traumatic edema.
   C. lymphedema.
   D. circulatory edema.

21. Which of the following statements best describes the functions of lymph nodes?

   A. filters lymph of impurities and acts as primary site for immune responses
   B. filters blood and produces white blood cells
   C. absorbs edema and filters it of impurities
   D. stores lymph in case of severe trauma

22. The right lumbar and left bronchomediastinal lymphatic trunks both carry lymph into which deep duct?

   A. abdominopelvic
   B. thoracic
   C. right lymphatic
   D. left lymphatic

23. What statement best describes the location of the lymphatic terminus?

   A. just lateral and deep to the abdominal aorta
   B. 1/3 supraclavicular and lateral to the sternal head of the SCM
   C. submandibular and anterior to the SCM
   D. just lateral to the clavicular head of the SCM and 2/3 subclavian

11: The Lymphatic System   153

24. Why is it important that lymph nodes have more afferent vessels than efferent?

  A. Fewer efferent vessels means more balanced flow into lymphatic trunks and ducts.

  B. It assures that the node will not lose too many of its stored lymphocytes.

  C. This creates an internal pressure differential that facilitates filtration.

  D. It assures that the node can be rapidly filled once emptied.

25. Which lymphotome bypasses the axillary catchment and carries lymph into the supraclavicular watershed instead?

  A. left subclavian

  B. right pectoral

  C. medial arm

  D. lateral arm

12

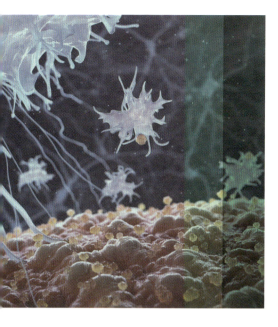

Immunity and Healing

Use this list to choose learning exercises that will help you expand and solidify your understanding of key topics. To test your knowledge, try the Review Quiz at the end of the chapter.

Key Topics	Exercise
• System or Immunity Terminology	1
• System Components and Lymphoid Tissue	2
• Nonspecific Immune Responses	3
• Specific Immune Responses	4
• Developing and Gaining Immunity	5 & 6

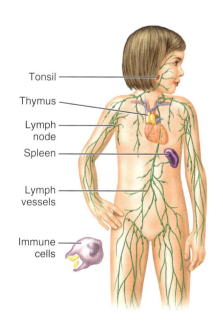

EXERCISE 1 • Immunity Crossword

Use this crossword to review and test your knowledge of the anatomy and physiology terms from Chapter 12.

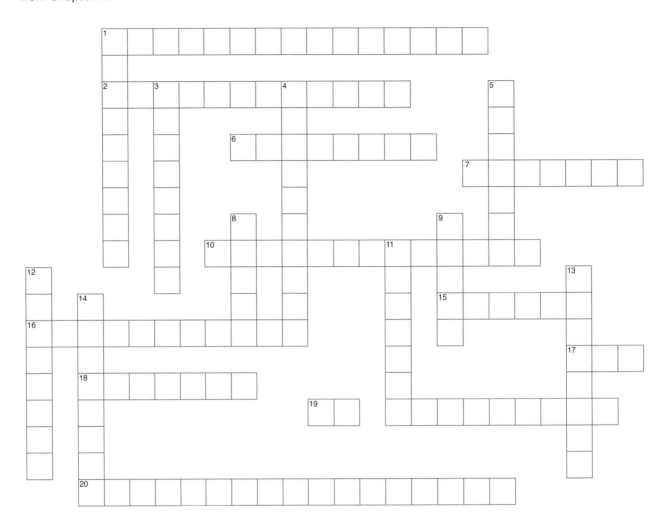

ACROSS

1. Specialized lymphocyte that inhibits or shuts down the body's specific immune response when it is no longer needed.
2. Disease resistance produced through the activation of T cells is _____ immunity.
6. Cell-signaling molecule.
7. Lymphoid tissues where lymphocytes are produced.
10. Small masses of lymphoid tissue located within the mucous membrane of the lower portion of the small intestine.
15. Any peptide molecule that binds to receptor proteins in the plasma membrane of target cells to stimulate cellular activity.
16. A plasma protein that binds iron when activated by a pathogen to make it unavailable to bacteria.
17. The study of the communication links between the nervous, endocrine, immune, and digestive systems.
18. Antibody-mediated immunity is also known as _____ immunity.
19. A group of general body defenses that are not directed at any particular pathogen; innate immune defense.
20. Disease resistance obtained without medical intervention is called _____ _____ immunity.

DOWN

1. The lymph nodes, spleen, and MALTs are considered this type of lymphoid tissue.
3. Any tissue that contains mature lymphocytes.
4. Cytokine that inhibits the spread of viral infection from infected to uninfected body cells.
5. A minute organism, including many types of pathogens such as bacteria and viruses.
8. Elevated core body temperature.
9. Specialized lymphocyte involved in antibody-mediated immunity.
11. Any substance that elicits a specific immune response.
12. A plasma protein released by plasma B cells that can bind with an antigen to neutralize or kill it; immunoglobulin.
13. Synonym for specific immune response.
14. Disease-causing agent such as bacteria, virus, allergen, or microbe.

EXERCISE 2 • Lymphoid Tissues

Match each of the following with its description. Then, use two different colors to highlight and distinguish the primary from the secondary lymphoid tissues.

_____ **1.** Red bone marrow

_____ **2.** Lymph node

_____ **3.** Spleen

_____ **4.** Thymus

_____ **5.** Tonsils

_____ **6.** Peyer's patches

_____ **7.** Appendix

_____ **8.** Adenoids

A. MALTs located in the mouth and throat

B. Filters blood, stores and releases lymphocytes

C. Filters lymph, stores and releases lymphocytes

D. Site of T lymphocyte maturation

E. MALTs in lower small intestine

F. Also known as the pharyngeal tonsils

G. Site of lymphocyte formation

H. Small twisted tube attached to the cecum

EXERCISE 3 • Nonspecific Immune Defenses

The nonspecific or **1.** _____ immune defenses of the body are a group of

2. _____ responses, that are neither stimulated by, nor directed toward,

3. _____ of pathogen or foreign invader.

For each nonspecific defense listed, provide a general description and specific examples where appropriate. The first bullet has been completed to get you started. If you need to refresh your memory, refer to Table 12.1 in your textbook.

• Physical barriers—Mechanical barriers such as the skin and mucous membranes that physically block

  microbes from entering the body

• Chemical barriers _____

_____

_____

• Internal antimicrobial proteins_____

_____

_____

• Phagocytes_____

_____

_____

• Natural killer cells_____

_____

_____

• Inflammation_____

_____

_____

• Fever _____

_____

_____

EXERCISE 4 • Specific Immune Responses

Specific or **1.** _____ immune responses are acquired over time through **2.** _____ to specific pathogens. These immune defenses involve **3.** _____ and _____ lymphocyte responses to **4.** _____ pathogenic agents, each with a recognizable chemical marker or **5.** _____ that identifies it as a **6.** _____ _____ and stimulates an **7.** _____ _____. For each unique **8.** _____ there is a lymphocyte with a corresponding **9.** _____ _____ on its plasma membrane. The response initiated by **10.** _____ cells is an **11.** _____ _____ or humoral response, while that initiated by **12.** _____ cells is a **13.** _____ _____ response. In most cases, both specific immune responses are stimulated by any particular pathogen.

Label the diagram to illustrate the specific immune responses. Answers may be either a component or a process. If you need to refresh your memory, refer to Figure 12.7 in the textbook.

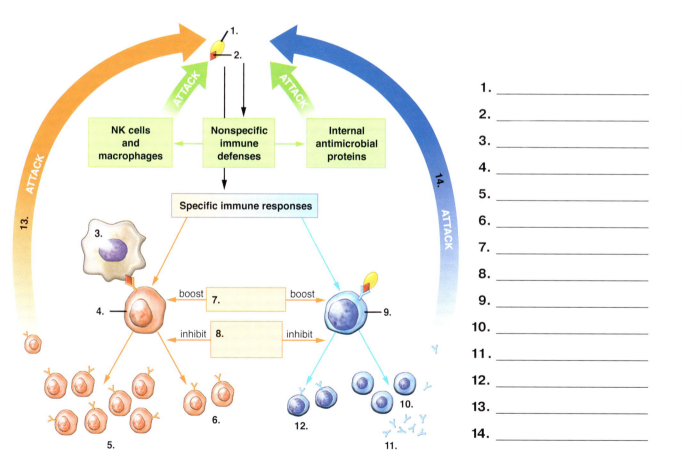

1. _____
2. _____
3. _____
4. _____
5. _____
6. _____
7. _____
8. _____
9. _____
10. _____
11. _____
12. _____
13. _____
14. _____

12: Immunity and Healing   159

EXERCISE 5 • A Story of Immunity

Taking the steps of a physiologic process and turning them into a story can help with understanding and recall. In addition, writing the story can be a creative way to review and organize information either individually or together as a group. The following provides one example of how a story about the body's immune response might begin. Have fun completing this story, or if you are not inspired by this beginning, write a different story altogether.

Once upon a time, there was a small and prosperous village called Wellsville. This village was often visited by artisans, peddlers, and tradesmen of nearby towns with whom they exchanged goods and services. One foggy day, a stranger wearing a cloak and carrying a staff with strange markings upon it arrived at the walls of Wellsville seeking entrance into the town. . . .

EXERCISE 6 • Gaining Immunity

Mark the following statements about naturally and artificially acquired immunity as T for true and F for false.

_____ **1.** Being immune to chicken pox after having it as a child is an example of naturally acquired immunity.

_____ **2.** Immunizations are examples of artificially acquired immunity.

_____ **3.** Immunity gained through actually having a disease like mumps is considered passively acquired natural immunity.

_____ **4.** A mother passing immunity to her infant through nursing is considered an active form of naturally acquired immunity.

_____ **5.** Getting a tetanus shot is an example of artificially acquired passive immunity.

_____ **6.** Getting an annual flu shot is an example of naturally acquired passive immunity.

_____ **7.** After children have measles, they have a lifelong immunity to the disease through naturally acquired active immunity.

_____ **8.** A polio vaccination is an example of artificially acquired active immunity.

REVIEW QUIZ

Immunity and Healing

Multiple Choice: Select the one best answer.

1. What is the name for the group of specialized white blood cells that are considered the primary immune cells?
   A. leukocytes
   B. primary lymphoids
   C. lymphocytes
   D. immunocytes

2. Which of these is classified as a primary lymphoid organ or tissue?
   A. lymph nodes
   B. spleen
   C. Peyer's patches
   D. red bone marrow

3. A _____ is a lymphocyte that is produced and matures in the bone marrow.
   A. MALT cell
   B. B cell
   C. T cell
   D. suppressor cell

4. Which of the sets of tonsils is also known as adenoids?
   A. lingual
   B. pharyngeal
   C. palatine
   D. nasal

5. Chemical barriers of the body include the pH of the skin and
   A. acidity of gastric juices.
   B. aldosterone release.
   C. peptide secretion.
   D. chemotaxis.

6. Another term for nonspecific immune defenses is
   A. innate immune defenses.
   B. physical immune defenses.
   C. general acquired immunity.
   D. internal immune environment.

7. Mucosa-associated lymphoid tissue (MALT) includes the tonsils and
   A. thymus.
   B. spleen.
   C. Peyer's patches.
   D. red bone marrow.

8. The four types of antimicrobial proteins are interferons, antimicrobial peptides, _____, and _____ .
   A. transferrins; complement proteins
   B. wandering macrophages; long-chain peptides
   C. neutrophils; macrophages
   D. antimicrobial lipids; transferrins

9. Where are lymphocytes initially produced?
   A. thymus
   B. red bone marrow
   C. lymph nodes
   D. spleen

10. What is the function of antimicrobial proteins?
    A. maturation of T cells in thymus
    B. provide the first line of internal nonspecific defense
    C. activate killer and helper T cells
    D. release specific immune enzymes that cause cytolysis of microbes

11. What are the two physical barriers that are key to our nonspecific immune defenses?
    A. serous and mucous membranes
    B. diaphragm and thoracic inlet
    C. the skin and teeth
    D. epidermis of skin and mucous membranes

12. What term is used to describe the process of phagocytes migrating to the site of infection in response to chemical signals released from cells in the area?
    A. cytolysis
    B. phagocytosis
    C. chemotaxis
    D. phagocytic migration

13. Which lymphocytes produce antibodies?
    A. memory T cells
    B. suppressor B cells
    C. NK cells
    D. plasma cells

14. What is another term for antibody?
    A. antigen
    B. allergen
    C. immunoglobulin
    D. interferon

162   REVIEW GUIDE

15. Which of the following are important processes of the general immune defense called inflammation?

   A. vasoconstriction and chemotaxis
   B. cytolysis and margination
   C. vasodilation and phagocytosis
   D. activation of B and T cells

16. Which of these antimicrobial proteins prevents bacterial proliferation by binding with iron in cells so it is not available to the microbe?

   A. interleukins
   B. inteferons
   C. complements
   D. transferrins

17. Which lymphocytes are involved in antibody-mediated immune responses?

   A. NK cells
   B. B lymphocytes
   C. helper T cells
   D. T lymphocytes

18. What are the two key characteristics that distinguish specific immune responses from general?

   A. It is always direct cell to cell and a body-wide process.
   B. All lymphoid tissues are involved and each has a specific job to do.
   C. It is an antigen-specific response and creates an immune memory.
   D. There is naturally acquired and artificially acquired specific immunity.

19. What is the function of suppressor T cells?

   A. inhibit and stop the immune response process once the challenge has passed
   B. stimulate NK cells to release antigen-suppressing enzymes
   C. inhibit the production of viral toxins
   D. monitor and regulate all T lymphocyte activity

20. What happens to antigens when antibodies attach to them?

   A. They are expelled via ciliary action.
   B. They are rendered ineffective.
   C. They get clumped together for NK cell destruction.
   D. Their nucleus is ruptured.

21. Which of these is an example of artificially acquired *active* immunity?

   A. transmission of antibodies from mother to child
   B. being exposed to a disease in childhood
   C. receiving injections of immunoglobulin
   D. vaccinations

22. Psychoneuroimmunology studies have clearly described two key communication networks, the autonomic nervous system and

   A. a system of neuroendocrine enzymes.
   B. a network of communication peptides called ligands.
   C. links between immune cells and neurofascial neurons.
   D. the endo-enteric nervous system.

23. Another term for antibody-mediated immunity is

   A. antigen-antibody response.
   B. antibody rush.
   C. humoral immunity.
   D. antigen-specific responses.

24. What special immune cells travel to the site of infection and directly destroy the foreign invader?

   A. cytotoxic T cells
   B. suppressor T cells
   C. memory B cells
   D. helper T cells

25. Which method of immunity acquisition is it when immunization delivers antibodies to provide immediate but short-term immunity?

   A. naturally acquired active
   B. naturally acquired passive
   C. artificially acquired active
   D. artificially acquired passive

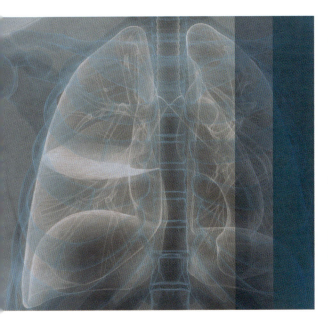

13

The Respiratory System

Use this list to choose learning exercises that will help you expand and solidify your understanding of key topics. To test your knowledge, try the Review Quiz at the end of the chapter.

Key Topics	Exercise
• System Terminology	1
• Primary System Structures, Divisions, and Functions	2–4, 8
• Muscles of Ventilation	5
• Physiology of Respiration	6 & 7

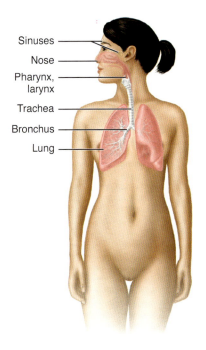

EXERCISE 1 • Respiratory System Crossword

Use this crossword to review and test your knowledge of the general anatomy and physiology terms from Chapter 13.

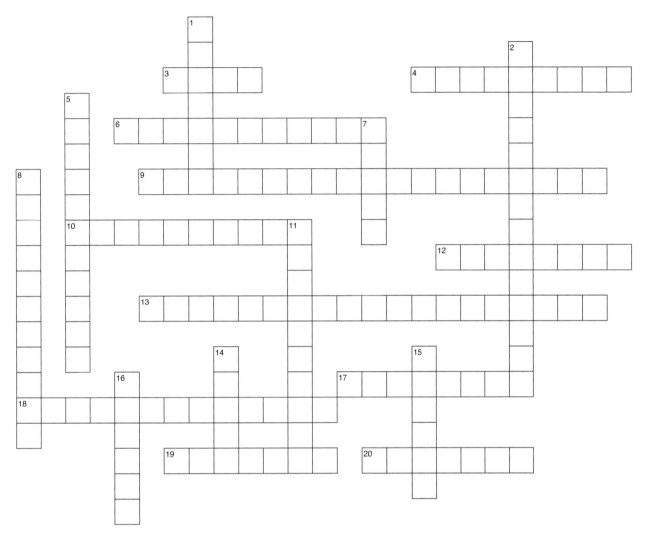

ACROSS

3 Respiratory regions are found in the medulla oblongata and _____.
4 Primary muscle of respiration.
6 Movement of air into and out of the lungs.
9 Formed by the alveolar and capillary walls.
10 Smallest air passageway of the bronchial tree.
12 Air sac in the lungs at the end of the bronchial tree.
13 Gas exchange between the air in the alveoli of the lungs and the bloodstream.
17 Muscles of respiration that insert on the 1st and 2nd ribs.
18 Primary method of transporting oxygen in the blood.
19 Passageway for air and food between the nose and larynx.
20 Nerve that innervates the diaphragm.

DOWN

1 Space between the vocal cords of the larynx.
2 Type of receptors that sense changes in oxygen and carbon dioxide blood levels.
5 Most CO_2 is converted into _____ ions for transport back to the lungs.
7 Nostrils.
8 Exchange of oxygen and carbon dioxide across the respiratory or cell membrane.
11 Expelling air from the lungs; expiration.
14 These structures beat upward and help remove particulate matter from air passages.
15 A serous membrane that lines the thoracic cavity and surrounds the lungs.
16 Cartilage and bony divider that separates the nasal cavity.

EXERCISE 2 • Respiratory Structures

Color the diagram of the respiratory system and label each of the specific structures. If you need to refresh your memory, refer to Figure 13.1 in the textbook.

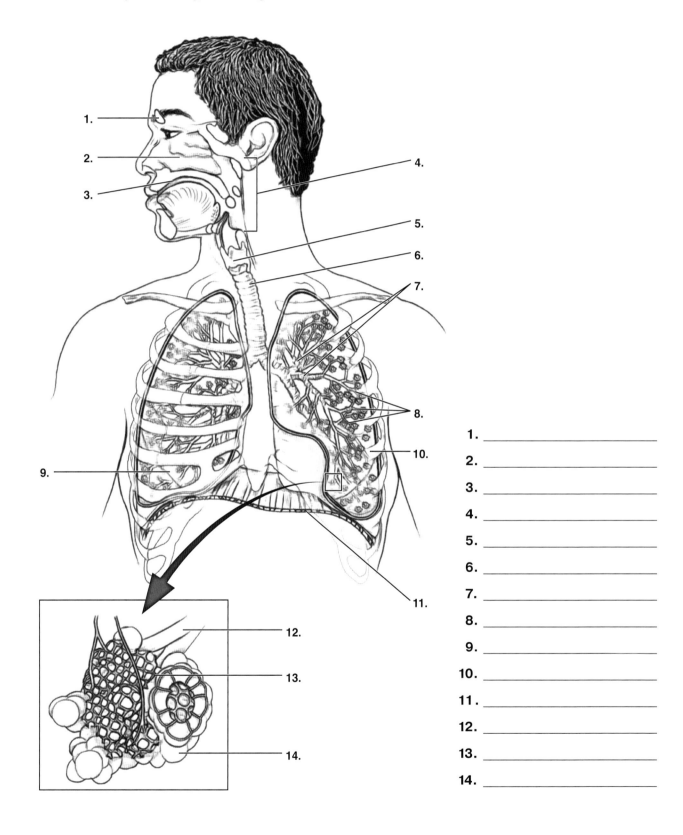

1. _____
2. _____
3. _____
4. _____
5. _____
6. _____
7. _____
8. _____
9. _____
10. _____
11. _____
12. _____
13. _____
14. _____

EXERCISE 3 • Matching Respiratory Organs

Match each of the respiratory structures with its proper location or function.

_____ **1.** Pharynx

_____ **2.** Nasal conchae

_____ **3.** Sinuses

_____ **4.** Trachea

_____ **5.** Lungs

_____ **6.** Alveoli

_____ **7.** Bronchioles

_____ **8.** Primary bronchi

_____ **9.** Pleura

_____ **10.** Larynx

_____ **11.** Respiratory membrane

_____ **12.** Respiratory cilia

A. Windpipe; passageway for air from pharynx to the bronchial tree

B. Hair-like projections in the respiratory mucosa that help trap small inhaled particles

C. Voice box; situated between the pharynx and trachea

D. Throat or posterior region of the mouth; serves as a common passageway for food and air

E. Scroll-shaped bony shelves in the nasal cavity that "ruffle" air to enhance olfaction and help humidify it

F. The first branches of the trachea that carry air into the lungs

G. Serous membrane that produces a lubricating fluid to decrease resistance for lung expansion

H. Mucous membrane–lined cavities in the frontal, maxillary, and ethmoid bones that humidify and warm air

I. Smallest branches of the bronchial tree

J. A thin membrane formed by the alveolar and capillary walls; produces surfactant to keep alveoli open

K. The largest organs of the respiratory system that fill the thoracic cavity on either side of the heart

L. Tiny air sacs; where respiration occurs

EXERCISE 4 • Upper or Lower Respiratory Tract

*Identify the following structures with a **U** if they are a part of the upper respiratory tract or an **L** if part of the lower respiratory tract.*

_____ **1.** Alveolar duct

_____ **2.** Respiratory membrane

_____ **3.** Lungs

_____ **4.** Trachea

_____ **5.** Larynx

_____ **6.** Primary bronchi

_____ **7.** Pharynx

_____ **8.** Epiglottis

_____ **9.** Sinuses

_____ **10.** Nasal conchae

EXERCISE 5 • Muscles of Ventilation

Place each of the muscles listed below on the table provided according to their location and/or action on the rib cage. Also, identify each as either a muscle of inhalation or exhalation by placing it in the correct column. Note that this will leave eight cells blank on the table. If you need to review the information about muscles of ventilation, check Figure 13.9 in the textbook.

Diaphragm	Rectus abdominis
External intercostals	Scalenes
Internal intercostals	Serratus anterior
Pectoralis minor	Sternocleidomastoid

DESCRIPTION	INHALATION	EXHALATION
The fiber direction of these short muscles between the ribs elevates the rib cage as a whole when they contract.	1.	
Contraction causes this muscle to flatten and increase the size of the rib cage.	2.	
This muscle's attachment to the sternum and lower ribs makes it depress the rib cage.	3.	
Contraction of these muscles pulls down on each individual rib, which depresses the rib cage as a whole.	4.	
These small muscles elevate the first two pairs of ribs when they contract.	5.	
Contraction of this muscle expands the rib cage laterally.	6.	
Contraction of this muscle helps elevate ribs 3 through 5.	7.	
Although it is a prime mover in rotation and flexion of the head, contraction of this muscle assists in ventilation by elevating the sternum and clavicle.	8.	

EXERCISE 6 • Respiration

Respiration is the physiologic process of **1.** _____.

This gaseous exchange takes place in two locations:

· **2.** _____

· **3.** _____

External respiration is the **4.** _____ while

5. _____ _____ is the gas exchange that occurs between the blood and body

tissues. The method of exchange is **6.** _____, and the gases are transported by binding to the

7. _____ on red blood cells, or as a dissolved substance in **8.** _____.

O_2 is transported through the blood as **9.** _____. CO_2 is transported through the

blood in three ways: approximately 80% of CO_2 is transported by converting it to **10.** _____

while the other 20% is transported either as **11.** _____ or as a dissolved gas.

170   REVIEW GUIDE

EXERCISE 7 • Respiration and Circulation

Color and label the diagram illustrating respiration and the circulation of blood to supply the body with oxygen and eliminate carbon dioxide. Be sure to draw in the arrows showing what direction the gases are moving. If you need to refresh your memory, refer to Figure 13.10 in the textbook.

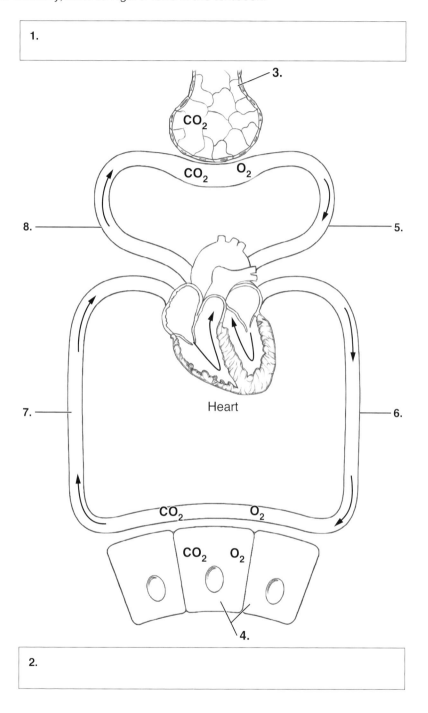

1. _____
2. _____
3. _____
4. _____
5. _____
6. _____
7. _____
8. _____

13: The Respiratory System

EXERCISE 8 • Building a Model of a Lung

In order to understand how the changing size of the thoracic cavity impacts the pressure and movement of air into and out of the lungs, build this simple model. For each model, you will need the following:

1- or 2-liter plastic pop bottle

Rigid plastic straw

Two balloons

One rubber band

Modeling clay

Scissors

Directions:

1. Cut the bottom off the plastic pop bottle. This will serve as the top and sides of the thoracic cavity.

2. Use the rubber band to fasten one balloon to the bottom of the straw.

3. Position the straw in the neck of the bottle so that the balloon hangs within the bottle. Create an airtight seal around the straw using a clump of modeling clay.

4. Cut off the top of the second balloon and then stretch it across the bottom of the plastic bottle. This flexible bottom will represent the diaphragm.

5. Now, to inflate your "lung," simply pinch the center of the "diaphragm" and slowly pull downward. As the "thoracic cavity" expands, notice that the "lung" attached to the end of the straw inflates.

REVIEW QUIZ

The Respiratory System

Multiple Choice: Select the one best answer.

1. The functions of the respiratory system are to provide oxygen for cellular activity, remove carbon dioxide, and
   A. provide a general immune response.
   B. provide moisture for digestive processes that occur in the mouth.
   C. help regulate temperature and fluid balance by eliminating heat and water.
   D. carry out the gustatory and olfactory general sensory functions.

2. What respiratory system structure serves as the site for the exchange of oxygen and carbon dioxide?
   A. oral cavity
   B. nasopharynx
   C. bronchioles
   D. alveoli

3. What is the function of the epiglottis?
   A. prevent food from entering the trachea during swallowing
   B. open the glottis to air as we inhale
   C. warm and moisten air before entering the trachea
   D. trap and expel pathogens that make it past the cilia in the nose

4. What is a functional purpose of the nose and sinuses?
   A. trap pathogens and control air volume
   B. warm and moisten air before it enters lungs
   C. balance the pH of the air
   D. provide an easy method of discharging mucus from the system

5. Which of these structures is a part of the lower respiratory tract?
   A. nasal cavity
   B. larynx
   C. trachea
   D. pharynx

6. Which respiratory structure houses the structures of voice production in addition to functioning as a passageway for air?
   A. pharynx
   B. sinus
   C. larynx
   D. trachea

7. What is the anatomical name for the structure commonly called the windpipe?
   A. nasopharynx
   B. laryngopharynx
   C. larynx
   D. trachea

8. Which term describes the process of moving air into and out of the lungs?
   A. ventilation
   B. respiration
   C. inspiration
   D. pulmonary process

9. The exchange of oxygen and carbon dioxide that occurs between the air and capillaries inside the lungs is called
   A. ventilation.
   B. internal respiration.
   C. external respiration.
   D. exhalation.

10. What transport mechanism is used for the exchange of oxygen and carbon dioxide between the lungs, blood, and body tissues?
    A. osmosis
    B. active transport
    C. filtration
    D. diffusion

11. Which of these statements correctly describes the gas exchange of external respiration?
    A. Oxygen moves out of the blood and carbon dioxide moves into it.
    B. Carbon dioxide and oxygen move into the blood.
    C. Carbon dioxide moves into the lungs and oxygen moves into the blood.
    D. Active transport moves oxygen into the tissues and carbon dioxide into blood.

12. What change occurs in the thoracic cavity when the diaphragm contracts?
    A. decreases in size
    B. increases in size
    C. the rib cage elevates
    D. the rib cage is depressed

13: The Respiratory System

13. Which of these skeletal muscles is considered *the* primary muscle of inspiration?

   A. diaphragm
   B. internal intercostals
   C. pectoralis minor
   D. scalenes

14. How is oxygen transported in the blood?

   A. as a dissolved gas in the plasma
   B. O_2 binds with plasma proteins
   C. as oxyhemoglobin on red blood cells
   D. as part of bicarbonate ions

15. The respiratory centers of the brain respond to stimulus from which types of receptors?

   A. nociceptors and mechanoreceptors
   B. stretch receptors and Golgi bodies
   C. thermoreceptors and chemoreceptors
   D. chemoreceptors and stretch receptors

16. Which condition provides the strongest stimulus to inhale?

   A. low levels of oxygen in the blood
   B. filling the lungs with air
   C. high levels of oxygen in the lungs
   D. high blood levels of carbon dioxide

17. Where are the chemoreceptors for breathing located?

   A. inside the walls of bronchioles and alveoli
   B. on outer surface of the pleural and respiratory membrane
   C. inside the walls of the carotid and aortic arteries
   D. on the cell membrane of red blood cells

18. How is *most* carbon dioxide transported in blood?

   A. as carbaminohemoglobin on red blood cells
   B. as bicarbonate ions
   C. by binding with hemoglobin
   D. via the plasma proeteins

19. Carbaminohemoglobin is formed during

   A. ventilation.
   B. external respiration.
   C. internal respiration.
   D. pulmonary obstruction.

20. Which nerves are the primary innervations for the muscles of ventilation?

   A. intercostal and phrenic
   B. vagus and thoracic
   C. intercostal and vagus
   D. phrenic and hepatic

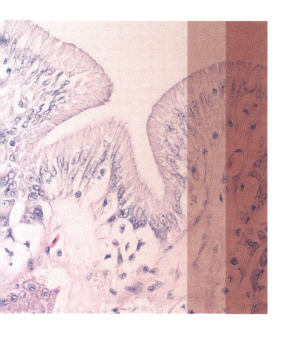

14

The Digestive System

Use this list to choose learning exercises that will help you expand and solidify your understanding of key topics. To test your knowledge, try the Review Quiz at the end of the chapter.

Key Topics	Exercise
• System Terminology	1
• The Divisions and Primary Organs of the System	2 & 3
• Layers of the GI Tract	4
• System Functions	5 & 6
• Metabolism and Nutrients	7

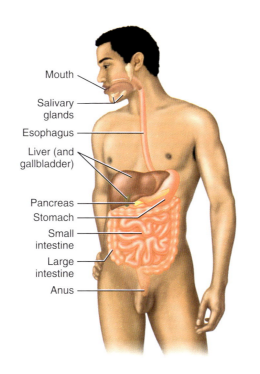

EXERCISE 1 • Digestive System Crossword

Use this crossword to review and test your knowledge of the general anatomy and physiology terms from Chapter 14.

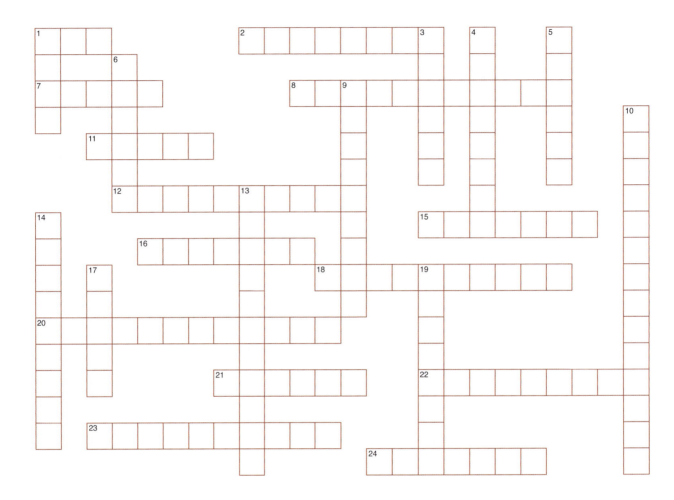

ACROSS

1. Baseline energy needed by the body to support basic life functions.
2. Initial segment of the small intestine.
7. Organ that secretes bile, stores fat and sugar as energy resources, and filters out toxins from blood.
8. The process of chewing.
11. The longest segment of the large intestine.
12. Assimilation of nutrients through the digestive tract into the blood is called _____.
15. Enzyme that digests starch.
16. The complex neuronal network that controls the secretions and smooth muscle contractions of the GI tract is the _____ nervous system.
18. Elimination of feces through the anus.
20. Mechanical digestive process that mixes and churns chyme in the SI.
21. Circular folds in the lining of the small intestine that increase the surface area for absorption.
22. The act of eating or taking in food or liquids.
23. Chewing is an example of this type of digestion.
24. Lower portion of the stomach.

DOWN

1. A fat emulsifier produced by the liver and stored in the gallbladder.
3. Innermost tissue layer of the digestive tract.
4. As a general function, movement within the GI tract is referred to as _____.
5. The upper portion of an organ such as the stomach.
6. Synonym for the visceral peritoneum.
9. Smooth muscle ring that controls the flow of substances through or out of the GI tract.
10. Large fatty extension (apron) of the peritoneum.
13. Wave-like muscular contraction that propels food through the GI tract.
14. The process of breaking down food so that nutrients can be absorbed.
17. Specialized folds in the lining of the stomach that allow it to distend.
19. The action of HCl in the stomach is considered an example of this type of digestion.

EXERCISE 2 • Gastrointestinal Tract Versus Accessory Organs and Functions

Mark each of the items listed as being either an accessory (A) or gastrointestinal (GI) tract organ or function.

_____ **1.** Absorption of nutrients

_____ **2.** Pancreas

_____ **3.** Stomach

_____ **4.** Esophagus

_____ **5.** Production and secretion of bile

_____ **6.** Liver

_____ **7.** Peristalsis

_____ **8.** Gallbladder

_____ **9.** Pharynx

_____ **10.** Secretion of amylase, lipase, and trypsin

_____ **11.** Absorption of water

_____ **12.** Secretion of hydrochloric acid

_____ **13.** Remove toxins and most medications from blood

EXERCISE 3 • Digestive System Organs

Color and label the diagrams of the digestive system. If you need to refresh your memory, refer to Figures 14.2, 14.8, and 14.11 in the textbook.

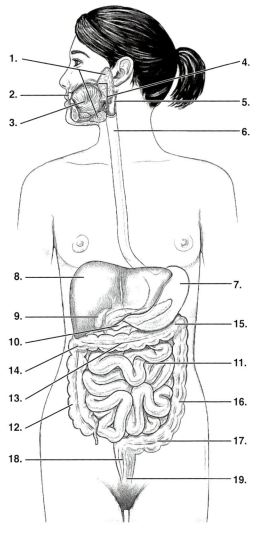

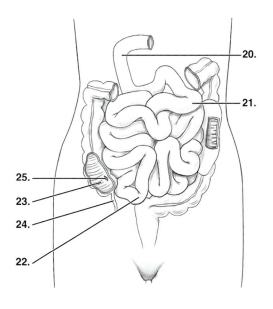

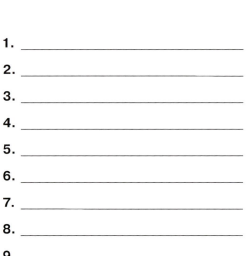

1. _____
2. _____
3. _____
4. _____
5. _____
6. _____
7. _____
8. _____
9. _____

10. _____
11. _____
12. _____
13. _____
14. _____
15. _____
16. _____
17. _____
18. _____
19. _____
20. _____
21. _____
22. _____
23. _____
24. _____
25. _____

EXERCISE 4 • Layers of the GI Tract

Complete the matching exercise to review or quiz your knowledge about the structure and function of each layer of the GI tract. Then, label the diagram below. If you need to refresh your memory, refer to Figure 14.3 in the textbook.

_____ 1. Mucosa
_____ 2. Submucosa
_____ 3. Muscularis
_____ 4. Serosa
_____ 5. Myenteric plexus
_____ 6. Peyer's patch
_____ 7. Mesentery
_____ 8. Submucosal plexus
_____ 9. Circular layer
_____ 10. Longitudinal layer

A. Propels food forward through the digestive tract
B. Visceral peritoneum
C. Double fold of peritoneum that supports SI
D. Includes motor neurons that control muscularis
E. Includes motor neurons that control mucosal secretions
F. MALT found in the intestines
G. Contains receptors that sense contents and distension of tract
H. Causes segmentation in the SI for mechanical digestion
I. Includes a third oblique layer in the stomach
J. Composed of areolar connective tissue

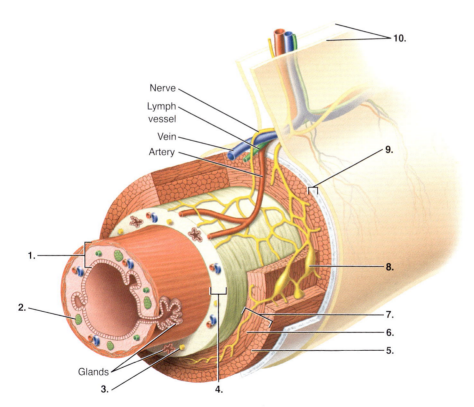

1. _____
2. _____
3. _____
4. _____
5. _____

6. _____
7. _____
8. _____
9. _____
10. _____

EXERCISE 5 • Functions of the Digestive System

Complete the table to summarize the functions of each organ of the digestive system. Note that ingestion and elimination have been omitted from the table since generally they only occur from one location; ingestion at the mouth and elimination from the anus. Also, notice that some boxes are empty because some organs carry out only one or two of the four functions listed. If you need to refresh your memory, refer back to Table 14.1 in the textbook. Remember that if you do not like tables, this same information can be organized using a mind map.

ORGAN	SECRETION	DIGESTION: MECHANICAL (M) AND CHEMICAL (C)	MOTILITY	ABSORPTION
Mouth and pharynx	Mucus	1. *M:* Chewing *C:*	2.	Sublingual medications
Salivary glands	3.			
Esophagus	Mucus		4.	
Stomach	5. Mucus plus . .	6. *M:* Mixing, grinding *C:* Breakdown of all foods via HCl and proteins by .	7. Gastric emptying and .	8. Some medications such as aspirin, and .
Small intestine	9. Mucus, sucrase, lactase, and maltase plus . Local hormones secretin and .	10. *M:* *C:* Breakdown of all nutrients with enzymes from the SI and pancreas, and fats with bile from the liver and gallbladder	11. Both . .	12. Water and medications plus . . .
Large intestine	13.		Peristalsis	14. Vitamin K and .

EXERCISE 6 • Diagram the Functions of the GI Tract

Sometimes a pictorial representation of information is more helpful than a table or mind map. For example, the schematic provided here can be used to summarize the functions of each organ of the GI tract. First, identify each of the organs labeled with a number on the schematic representation of the GI tract. Next, draw a line(s) from each function box to the region(s) of the tract where the function takes place. Finally, complete each function box by placing the number of each organ where the function occurs and providing a brief description. An example has been provided for you under mechanical digestion. Also, consider adding color to further visually organize the information, either by coloring each structure a different color and using it to highlight its place in each function box, or by color coding the functions and adding colored squiggles or layers to each organ where the function takes place.

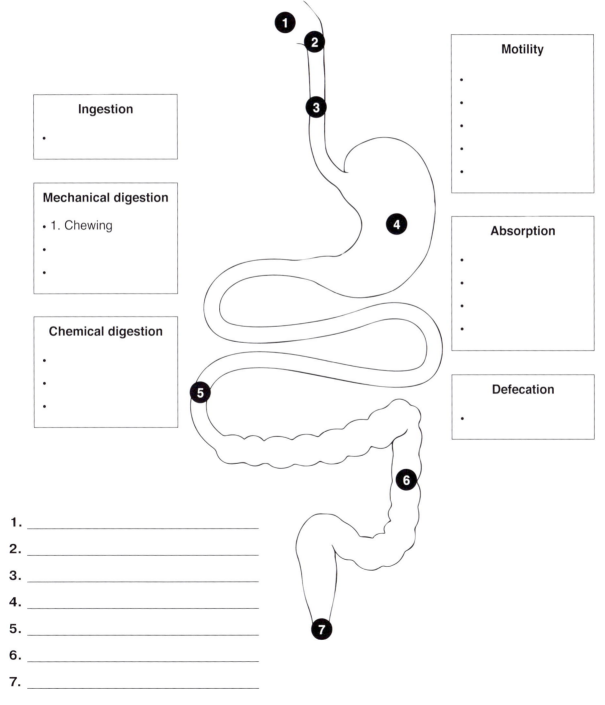

Ingestion
-

Mechanical digestion
- 1. Chewing
-
-

Chemical digestion
-
-
-

Motility
-
-
-
-
-

Absorption
-
-
-
-

Defecation
-

1. _____
2. _____
3. _____
4. _____
5. _____
6. _____
7. _____

14: The Digestive System   181

EXERCISE 7 • Metabolism and Nutrients

Metabolism refers to all the **1.** _____ _____ that occur within the body. It includes

2. _____ processes, in which complex molecules are formed from simpler ones, tissue is

created or **3.** _____, and molecules such as hormones, neurotransmitters, and ligands are

4. _____. Metabolism also includes **5.** _____ processes such as glycolysis and

the Krebs cycle, which break down complex molecules to **6.** _____ _____ .

All of these processes rely on the body's intake and assimilation of two general categories of nutrients through

the digestive system.

7. _____ are needed in large quantities to meet the body's tissue-building and energy

demands. They include:

- Carbohydrates that are absorbed as **8.** _____ molecules that can be easily catabolized for

   9. _____ via glycolysis and the Krebs cycle, or converted into **10.** _____ to

   be stored in skeletal muscle and the liver, or into **11.** _____ and stored as adipose tissue.

- **12.** _____ are absorbed as triglyceride molecules and broken into **13.** _____

   and _____ _____, which can be catabolized for energy. They are stored as

   14. _____ tissue.

- Proteins absorbed as **15.** _____ _____ can be converted in the

   16. _____ and catabolized to produce ATP, but they are the body's last choice for energy

   production. More importantly, these molecules are used for all types of **17.** _____

   _____ to make and repair tissue, and form **18.** _____.

19. _____ are only needed in small amounts by the body to maintain homeostasis and health.

These nutrients include:

- Vitamins that support normal metabolic function by **20.** _____.

- **21.** _____ that support homeostatic mechanisms including pH, fluid, and energy balance;

   are important components of **22.** _____ and _____ tissues; and serve as

   23. _____ .

While not technically a nutrient, **24.** _____ is also essential for cellular health and the

maintenance of homeostasis.

REVIEW QUIZ

The Digestive System

Multiple Choice: Select the one best answer.

1. Which of the six digestive processes is when food is broken down into usable molecules?
   - **A.** digestion
   - **B.** ingestion
   - **C.** secretion
   - **D.** motility

2. What is another term for the digestive process of elimination?
   - **A.** micturition
   - **B.** mechanical excretion
   - **C.** myenteric releasing
   - **D.** defecation

3. Which of these digestive organs are located in the upper right quadrant of the abdominopelvic cavity?
   - **A.** spleen and pancreas
   - **B.** liver and colon
   - **C.** liver and gallbladder
   - **D.** stomach and spleen

4. The outermost layer of the gastrointestinal tract is the serosa, also known as the
   - **A.** endosteum.
   - **B.** peritoneum.
   - **C.** smooth muscle layer.
   - **D.** submucosa.

5. Where does the chemical digestion of starch begin?
   - **A.** mouth
   - **B.** esophagus
   - **C.** small intestine
   - **D.** stomach

6. Where does the process of peristalsis begin?
   - **A.** pharynx
   - **B.** stomach
   - **C.** esophagus
   - **D.** small intestine

7. Where does the chemical digestion of protein begin?
   - **A.** mouth
   - **B.** stomach
   - **C.** small intestine
   - **D.** pancreas

8. Which of these is an accessory organ to digestion?
   - **A.** salivary glands
   - **B.** stomach
   - **C.** esophagus
   - **D.** small intestine

9. Besides elimination, what is the other function of the large intestine?
   - **A.** protein digestion
   - **B.** complete carbohydrate digestion
   - **C.** secretion of bicarbonates to neutralize acidic chyme
   - **D.** absorption of water

10. What is the name of the valve between the large and small intestines?
    - **A.** duodenal
    - **B.** esophageal
    - **C.** pyloric
    - **D.** ileocecal

11. Which two organs are retroperitoneal?
    - **A.** stomach and espohagus
    - **B.** pancreas and duodenum
    - **C.** jejunum and transverse colon
    - **D.** pancreas and gallbladder

12. What is the function of the greater omentum?
    - **A.** cover and protect the abdominal viscera
    - **B.** lubricate the peritoneum
    - **C.** insulate and cushion the abdominopelvic cavity
    - **D.** hold the blood supply for all organs in GI tract

13. What is the name for the point of intersection between the transverse and descending colon?
    - **A.** splenic flexure
    - **B.** transverso-inferior flexure
    - **C.** hepatic flexure
    - **D.** sigmoid flexure

14. What is the function of the enteric nervous system?
    - **A.** signaling the external sphincter of the anus for defecation
    - **B.** regulation of bile production and secretion
    - **C.** inhibition of ingestion
    - **D.** regulation of digestive secretions and motility

14: The Digestive System

15. Digestion of fats results in the production of what absorbable molecule?

   A. amino acid
   B. glycogen
   C. glucose
   D. triglyceride

16. What is the function of the lacteals?

   A. secrete lipase for fat digestion
   B. absorb fats from the small intestine
   C. remove water from the colon to compact particles into feces
   D. secrete amylase for carbohydrate digestion

17. The majority of digestion and absorption occurs in which organ?

   A. stomach
   B. pancreas
   C. small intestine
   D. large intestine

18. What process builds actin, myosin, and collagen?

   A. anabolism of amino acids
   B. catabolism of fatty acids
   C. anabolism of glycerol
   D. catabolism of lipids

19. Which of these is NOT part of the digestive juice secreted by the pancreas?

   A. peptidases
   B. bicarbonate
   C. lipase
   D. secretin

20. Which of these is NOT a function of the liver?

   A. secretion of bile
   B. storage of glycogen
   C. secretion of protein digestive enzymes
   D. filtering toxins from the blood

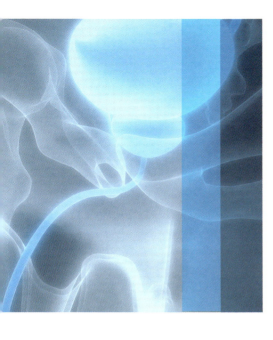

15

The Urinary System

Use this list to choose learning exercises that will help you expand and solidify your understanding of key topics. To test your knowledge, try the Review Quiz at the end of the chapter.

Key Topics	Exercise
• System Terminology	1
• Structures of the System	2
• Structure of Kidneys	3
• Structure and Processes of Nephrons	4 & 5
• The Kidney's Role in Fluid Management	6

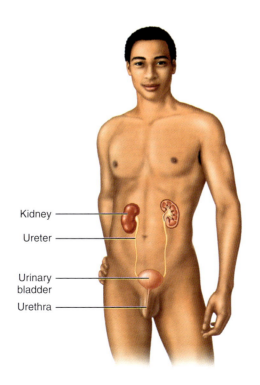

EXERCISE 1 • Urinary System Crossword

Use this crossword to review and test your knowledge of the general anatomy and physiology terms from Chapter 15.

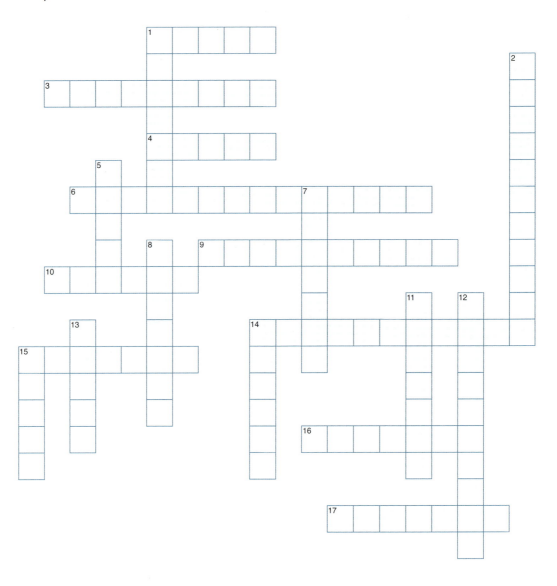

ACROSS

1. Liquid waste formed by the kidneys.
3. In this process, toxins, metabolic wastes, and unused ions and nutrients are moved out of the blood into the renal tubule.
4. Indentation in the kidney where the ureters, blood vessels, and nerves enter and exit the organ.
6. Initial portion of a nephron composed of the glomerulus and Bowman's capsule.
9. Wad of capillaries found in the nephron.
10. Region of the kidney where urine is collected before being passed into the ureter.
14. Stress initiates the RAA pathway because sympathetic stimulation leads to a decrease in renal _____.
15. Hollow organ that serves as a holding tank for urine.
16. The inner portion of the kidneys is called the renal _____.
17. Microscopic functional unit of the kidney.

DOWN

1. Narrow tube that carries urine from the bladder to the external environment.
2. Urination.
5. Pertaining to the kidneys.
7. These tubes connect the kidneys to the bladder.
8. Blood levels of essential electrolytes such as Na^+, K^+, H^+, and OH^- are all regulated by the _____.
11. Large fascial envelope that surrounds each kidney and attaches it to the abdominal wall.
12. The specific urine formation process that occurs in the renal corpuscle.
13. Small cup at the bottom of a renal pyramid that collects urine.
14. The renal _____ is the outer portion of the kidney.
15. The kidneys filter and cleanse this fluid through the process of urine formation.

EXERCISE 2 • Urinary System Organs

Color and label the diagram to identify the organs of the urinary system. Then, for each structural characteristic or function listed, place the letter of the organ described. Note that some organs are described in more than one way, so their letters will be used multiple times. If you need to refresh your memory, refer to Figure 15.1 in the textbook.

_____ 1. This organ carries urine from the kidneys to the bladder.
_____ 2. This organ has rugae for distension.
_____ 3. This organ helps to balance blood pH, electrolytes, and fluid volumes.
_____ 4. This organ is partially situated anterior to the twelfth rib.
_____ 5. This organ has two muscular sphincters that regulate elimination.
_____ 6. This organ's wall has three layers of smooth muscle.
_____ 7. These mucus-lined tubes are retroperitoneal.
_____ 8. This organ's function is affected by ADH and aldosterone.
_____ 9. This organ secretes the hormone calcitriol.
_____ 10. This organ releases renin in response to stress.

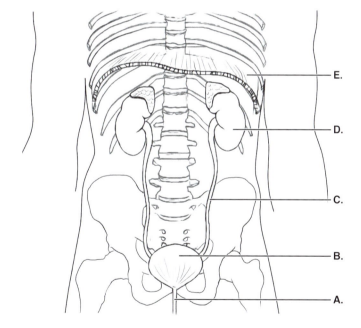

A. _____
B. _____
C. _____
D. _____
E. _____

EXERCISE 3 • Structure of the Kidneys

Color and label the diagram detailing the structure of the kidney. Provide a brief definition of each component identified. If you need to refresh your memory, refer to Figure 15.2 in the textbook.

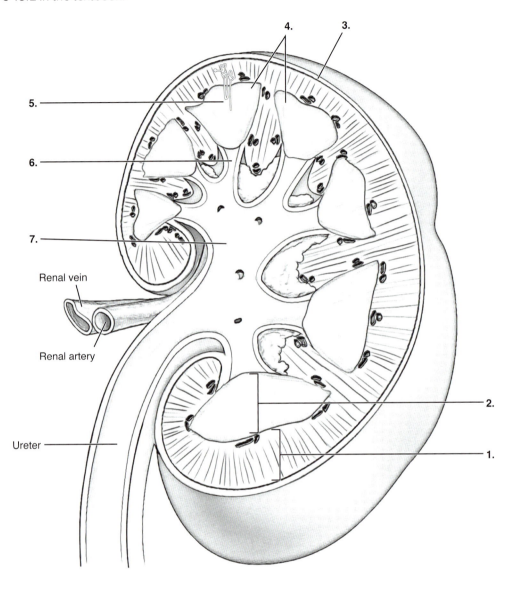

1. _____
2. _____
3. _____
4. _____
5. _____
6. _____
7. _____

EXERCISE 4 • Parts of a Nephron

Label the structural components of the nephron. You may want to look at the next exercise for some of the names of the structures, or if you need to refresh your memory, refer to Figure 15.5 in the textbook.

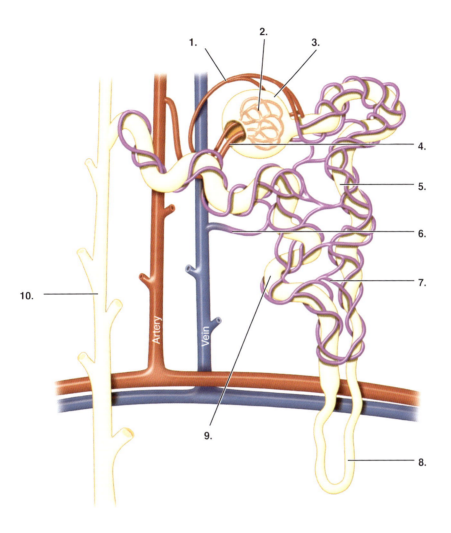

1. _____
2. _____
3. _____
4. _____
5. _____
6. _____
7. _____
8. _____
9. _____
10. _____

15: The Urinary System 189

EXERCISE 5 • Structure and Function of a Nephron

Match each of the structures and functions of a nephron to its proper description.

_____ **1.** Glomerulus

_____ **2.** Distal convoluted tubule

_____ **3.** Filtration

_____ **4.** Renal corpuscle

_____ **5.** Collecting duct

_____ **6.** Bowman's capsule

_____ **7.** Secretion

_____ **8.** Proximal convoluted tubule

_____ **9.** Reabsorption

_____ **10.** Peritubular capillaries

A. The first step in urine formation

B. Nephron segment where filtration occurs

C. The outer portion of the renal corpuscle

D. Where most reabsorption takes place

E. Process in which water, sodium, and other electrolytes move from the renal tubule into blood

F. Ball of capillaries inside the renal corpuscle

G. Network of blood vessels around the renal tubule for the exchange of fluid and substances between blood and urine

H. Elimination of ammonia, urea, and excess hydrogen ions from blood to urine

I. Site where fluid from several nephrons is concentrated into urine

J. Nephron segment where most secretion takes place

EXERCISE 6 • The Kidney's Role in Fluid Management

As the kidneys filter and cleanse the blood, they play a central role in managing the volume and composition of the blood. Use the mind map provided to record the kidney's role in fluid management. As your mind map expands, be sure to also consider the links between the itemized roles. For example, explore the connection between blood pressure and blood volume, or between blood pH and electrolytes.

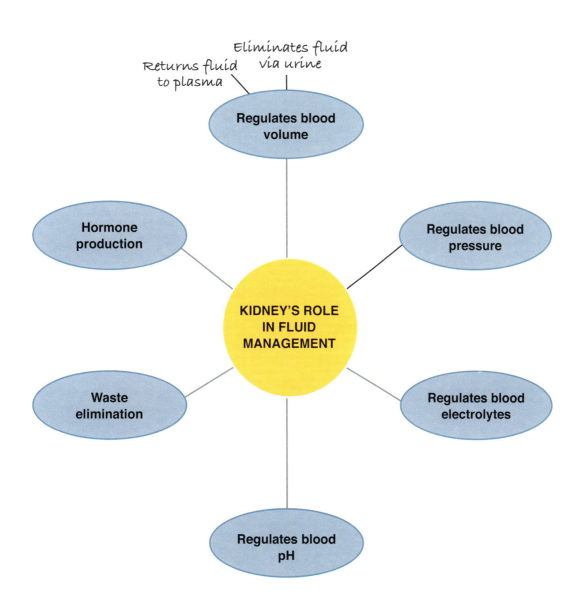

REVIEW QUIZ

The Urinary System

Multiple Choice: Select the one best answer.

1. The four components of the urinary system are kidneys, bladder,
   - A. urinary sphincters, and renal calyx.
   - B. glomerulus, and renal capsule.
   - C. ureters, and nephrons.
   - D. urethra, and ureters.

2. The functions of the urinary system include helping to regulate pH, blood pressure, and fluid volume, plus
   - A. secretion of hormones.
   - B. recycling worn out red blood cells.
   - C. removing metabolic waste from lymph.
   - D. lipid catabolism.

3. Which urinary organ serves as the site for urine storage?
   - A. kidneys
   - B. bladder
   - C. ureters
   - D. urethra

4. What is the difference between the ureters and urethra?
   - A. Ureters are in the kidneys and urethra is a tube that passes urine to external environment.
   - B. Ureters are more muscular tubes that move urine through peristalsis.
   - C. The urethra is more external than the ureters.
   - D. Ureters carry urine from kidneys to bladder and urethra goes from bladder to external environment.

5. Which of these is considered the functional unit of the urinary system?
   - A. glomerulus
   - B. nephron
   - C. renal medulla
   - D. renal cortex

6. What is the name of the outer section of tissue in the kidney?
   - A. renal cortex
   - B. renal medulla
   - C. renal hilus
   - D. renal tubule

7. What hormone secreted by the kidneys stimulates red blood cell production in bone marrow?
   - A. calcitriol
   - B. erythropoietin
   - C. aldosterone
   - D. glucocorticoids

8. What is the name for the bulbous portion of the nephron?
   - A. hilus
   - B. renal cortex
   - C. renal circularis
   - D. renal corpuscle

9. The expansion at the upper end of the ureter inside the kidney is called the
   - A. calyx.
   - B. pyramid.
   - C. pelvis.
   - D. internal ureter.

10. What two structures make up the renal corpuscle?
    - A. proximal and distal corpuscle
    - B. glomerulus and proximal tubule
    - C. renal and adipose capsule
    - D. Bowman's capsule and glomerulus

11. Where in the kidneys does the first step of urine formation occur?
    - A. renal corpuscle
    - B. renal medulla
    - C. loop of Henle
    - D. peritubular capillaries

12. During urine formation, the majority of secretion processes occur in which portion of the nephron?
    - A. proximal convoluted tubule
    - B. distal convoluted tubule
    - C. loop of Henle
    - D. collecting duct

13. Which urine formation process moves substances such as glucose and water out of the renal tubule and into the blood?
    - A. filtration
    - B. reabsorption
    - C. secretion
    - D. urine concentration

14. What is the name for the bundle of capillaries inside Bowman's capsule?

   A. glomerulus
   B. peritubular capillaries
   C. Bowman's capillaries
   D. renal corpuscle

15. What is the physiologic term for expelling urine from the body?

   A. elimination
   B. micturition
   C. mastication
   D. defecation

16. What is the normal concentration of water in urine?

   A. 10%
   B. 50%
   C. 95%
   D. 75%

17. Urine generally contains high concentrations of nitrogenous waste products such as urea, ammonia, and

   A. phosphates.
   B. uric acid.
   C. calcium bicarbonate.
   D. amino acid.

18. Where is the internal sphincter of the urinary system located?

   A. the junction between the kidney and ureter
   B. between the renal cortex and medulla
   C. the junction between the ureter and bladder
   D. at the more proximal end of the urethra

19. What structure in the urinary system is under voluntary muscle control?

   A. external sphincter
   B. internal sphincter
   C. Bowman's capsule
   D. urethra

20. What percentage of nephron filtrate is reabsorbed from the nephron back into the bloodstream?

   A. 25% to 30%
   B. 45% to 50%
   C. 73% to 75%
   D. 97% to 99%

15: The Urinary System   193

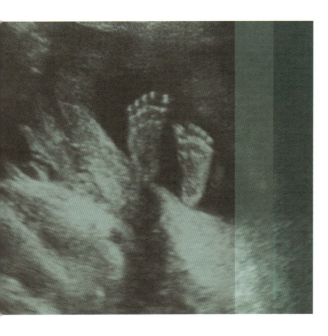

16

The Reproductive System

Use this list to choose learning exercises that will help you expand and solidify your understanding of key topics. To test your knowledge, try the Review Quiz at the end of the chapter.

Key Topics	Exercise
• System Terminology	1
• Common Characteristics of Male and Female Systems	2
• Male Components and Functions	3 & 4
• Female Components and Functions	5 & 6

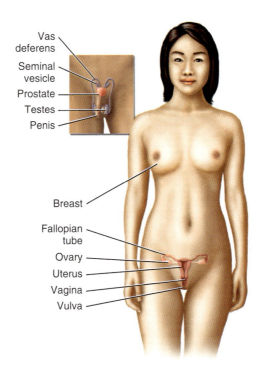

EXERCISE 1 • Reproductive System Crossword

Use this crossword to review and test your knowledge of the general anatomy and physiology terms from Chapter 16.

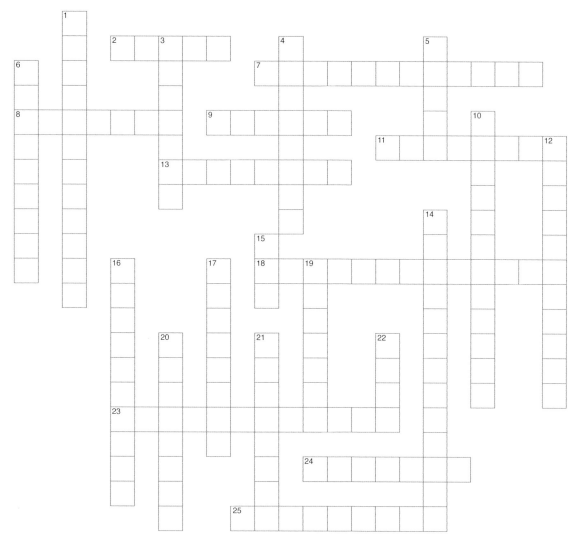

ACROSS

2 Male gamete.
7 Hormone produced by Leydig cells.
8 Passageway for both sperm and urine in males.
9 Fertilized egg.
11 The first menstrual period and beginning of the reproductive cycle.
13 Embryonic layer that differentiates to form the epidermis, nervous tissue, and sense organs.
18 Days 6 through 14 of the female reproductive cycle, when the endometrium thickens, is called the _____ phase.
23 Glandular mass formed from the follicle once the ovum has been discharged.
24 Gametes are produced through this cell division process.
25 Period of fetal development from conception until birth.

DOWN

1 Painful or difficult menstruation.
3 In the first stage of labor, the cervix dilates and _____ (thins and shortens).
4 Middle embryonic layer that differentiates to form muscle and connective tissues.
5 Thick, whitish fluid consisting of sperm and secretions from several accessory reproductive organs.
6 The expelling of an egg from the ovary.
10 Female steroid hormone that stimulates the development and maintenance of the endometrium.
12 Inner lining of the uterus that thickens and sloughs off with each menstrual cycle.
14 A synonym for conception; when sperm penetrates an egg.
15 A common condition for men over 50.
16 Multicelled mass of tissue that develops into an embryo.
17 The region between the mons pubis and anus in females, or the scrotum and anus in males.
19 Synonym for fallopian tube.
20 Hormone that stimulates the maturation of ova within the ovaries.
21 Specialized ring of cells surrounding an ovum.
22 Female gamete.

16: The Reproductive System

EXERCISE 2 • Mind Map of Common Characteristics

Complete the mind map by specifying the male and female reproductive features for each of the common characteristics identified. If you need to refresh your memory, refer to Table 16.1 in the textbook.

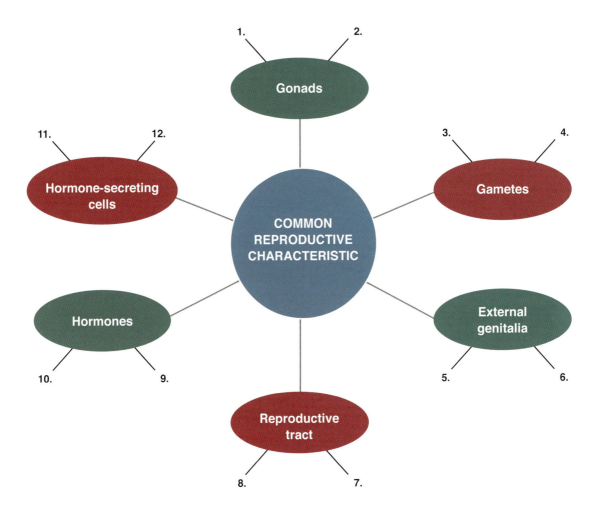

EXERCISE 3 • Male Pelvic Anatomy

Color and label the sagittal section to identify the structures of the male pelvic cavity. Highlight the labels of the reproductive components to help differentiate them from other pelvic structures. If you need to refresh your memory, refer to Figure 16.1 in the textbook.

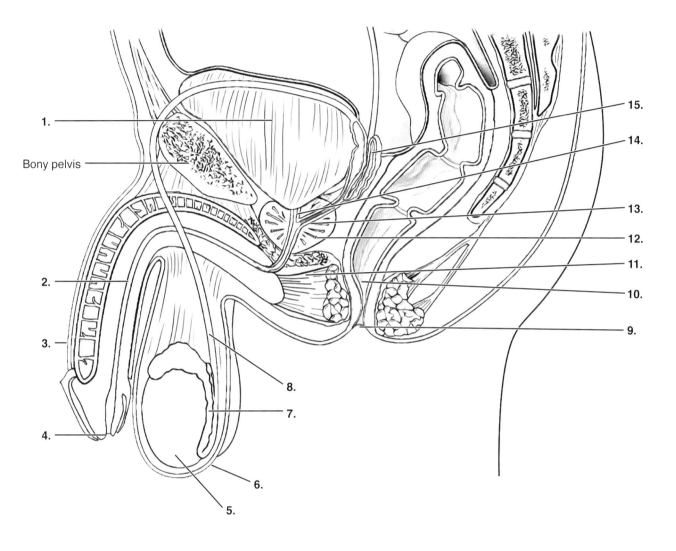

1. _____
2. _____
3. _____
4. _____
5. _____
6. _____
7. _____
8. _____
9. _____
10. _____
11. _____
12. _____
13. _____
14. _____
15. _____

EXERCISE 4 • Male Reproductive Structures and Functions

Match each of the structures in the male reproductive system with its function or key structural characteristic.

_____ **1.** Seminal vesicle

_____ **2.** Testes

_____ **3.** Vas deferens

_____ **4.** Seminiferous tubule

_____ **5.** Epididymis

_____ **6.** Ejaculatory duct

_____ **7.** Leydig cells

_____ **8.** Prostate gland

_____ **9.** Bulbourethral glands

A. Sperm mature, develop their motility and ability to fertilize in this structure

B. Sperm production and secretion of testosterone

C. Duct that carries sperm from the prostate to the urethra

D. Produce testosterone

E. Produces 60% of the fluid portion of semen

F. Secretes a milky fluid directly into the urethra to support sperm motility

G. Stores sperm for several months and carries it out of the scrotum to the spermatic cord

H. Produces mucus-like substance that lubricates the lining of the urethra to protect sperm during ejaculation

I. Male gonads that produce male gametes

EXERCISE 5 • Female Pelvic Anatomy

Color and label the sagittal section to identify the structures of the female pelvic cavity. Highlight the labels of the reproductive components to help differentiate them from other pelvic structures. If you need to refresh your memory, refer to Figure 16.3 in the textbook.

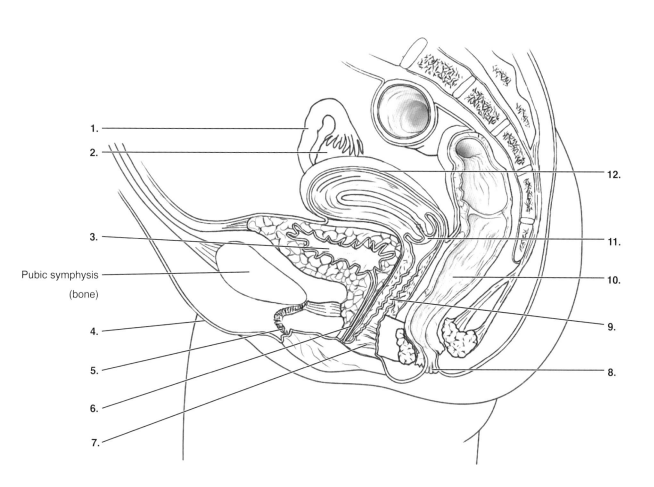

16: The Reproductive System 199

EXERCISE 6 • Female Reproductive Structures and Functions

Match each of the structures in the female reproductive system with its function or key structural characteristic.

_____ **1.** Follicle

_____ **2.** Corpus luteum

_____ **3.** Endometrium

_____ **4.** Fallopian tube

_____ **5.** Fimbriae

_____ **6.** Vagina

_____ **7.** Uterus

_____ **8.** Ovary

_____ **9.** Placenta

_____ **10.** Labia

A. Short muscular tube that carries eggs from the ovary to the uterus

B. Produces ova, estrogen, and progesterone

C. Blood-rich, protective membrane for the fetus

D. Canal between the cervix and exterior environment

E. Inner lining of the uterus that thickens and sloughs off with each menstrual cycle

F. Hormone-secreting, glandular mass formed from the follicle once the ovum has been discharged

G. Lateral tissue folds that surround the vaginal and urethral openings

H. Specialized ring of cells surrounding an ovum inside the ovaries

I. Finger-like projections off the fallopian tube that surround the ovaries to help "catch" the egg

J. Hollow, muscular organ that houses the developing fetus

REVIEW QUIZ

The Reproductive System

Multiple Choice: Select the one best answer.

1. Both the male and female reproductive systems share what four organizational and structural features?
   A. gonads, accessory organs, genitalia, hormonal control processes
   B. internal and external genitalia, gonads, onsite hormone production, neuroendocrine control
   C. gonads, hypothalamic hormonal production, gametes, number of accessory organs
   D. gametes, gonads, equal maturation rates of gametes, use positive feedback mechanisms

2. What is the definition of ovulation?
   A. production of the gametes in the gonads
   B. the secretion of fluids from testes and ovary
   C. expelling of an egg from the ovary
   D. the first stage in the gestation process

3. What male accessory gland is donut-shaped and encircles the upper urethra?
   A. bulbourethral
   B. spermatic
   C. seminal
   D. prostate

4. The joining of the genetic materials from sperm and egg is called
   A. day 1.
   B. fertilization.
   C. reproduction.
   D. implantation.

5. Which structure in the testes produces sperm?
   A. epididymis
   B. Leydig cells
   C. seminal vesicle
   D. seminiferous tubules

6. Which of the following structures secretes progesterone?
   A. follicle
   B. ovum
   C. corpus luteum
   D. fimbriae

7. Which of the following is NOT a part of the duct network that carries sperm?
   A. seminal vesicle
   B. epididymis
   C. vas deferens
   D. urethra

8. Which structure in the female reproductive system is also called the birth canal?
   A. uterus
   B. vagina
   C. oviducts
   D. fallopian tubes

9. At what stage of pregnancy is the term embryo applied?
   A. day one
   B. first week
   C. third week
   D. ninth week

10. The cervix is which region of the uterus?
    A. superior dome
    B. wide central zone
    C. narrow distal zone
    D. the muscular wall

11. Which hormone is responsible for building and maintaining the uterine lining?
    A. progesterone
    B. estrogen
    C. follicle-stimulating hormone
    D. luteinizing hormone

12. What is the function of the prostate gland?
    A. secretion of semen
    B. development of sperm
    C. initiating ejaculation
    D. secrete a milky fluid that prevents semen clotting

13. Where does fertilization of the egg generally occur?
    A. inside the fallopian tube
    B. inside the vagina
    C. at the entrance of the uterus
    D. at the junction between uterus and oviduct

16: The Reproductive System

14. During which days of the menstrual cycle does menstruation occur?

   A. 6 through 14

   B. 9 through 20

   C. 1 through 5

   D. 14 through 28

15. What is the name of the protective sac that encloses the testes?

   A. vas deferens

   B. spermatic sac

   C. seminal vesicle

   D. scrotum

Answer Key

Chapter 1

EXERCISE 1 Terminology Crossword

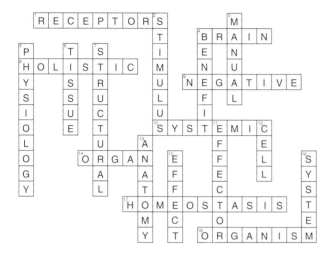

EXERCISE 2 Describing the Levels of Organization

1. Organism or Whole body
2. System = a group of organs working together
3. Organ = a group of tissues working together
4. Tissue = a group of like cells working together
5. Cell = smallest functional unit of the body
6. Chemicals = atoms and molecules, the building blocks of living matter

EXERCISE 5 Homeostasis Flow Chart

Integration center (bow tie shape) receives input from receptor, interprets information, and passes command to the effector

Stimulus (sunburst shape) change in the environment

Effector (rectangle) cells, tissue, or organs that respond to change

Receptor (oval) sense organ sensitive to specific type of stimulus

EXERCISE 6 Negative and Positive Feedback

1. Counteracts or reverses
2. Reinforces or sustains

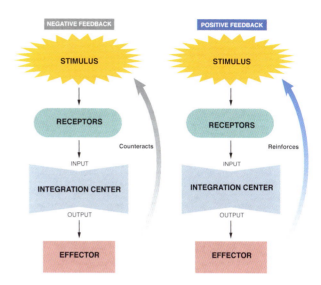

EXERCISE 7 Linking Body, Mind, and Spirit

The following are just examples. Your answers should reflect your own ideas, thoughts, and feelings.

TENSE:
  Body: tight and head aches
  Mind: scattered but alert
  Spirit: uptight and constricted

FEAR:
  Body: uptight and on alert
  Mind: worried and concerned
  Spirit: nervous and suspicious

JOY:
  Body: loose and energetic
  Mind: alert and creative
  Spirit: happy and content

EXERCISE 8 Benefits and Effects of Manual Therapy

1. B
2. E
3. E
4. B
5. E
6. B
7. B
8. E
9. E
10. E

Structural effects may include things such as releasing adhered connective tissue, while systemic effects may include loosening and softening tissues, reduction of edema, or enhanced local fluid flow.

Answer Key   203

EXERCISE 9 Manual Therapy Categories

1. Sliding/gliding style of work that uses a lubricant for a full-body session

2. Traditional massage, Wellness/health maintenance massage, Relaxation massage, Spa massage & Stress reduction massage

3. Stretching, loosening, or broadening

4. Improve range of motion (ROM); decrease pain

5. Any of the following: Active Release Techniques® (ART), Hellerwork®, Joint mobilization, Myofascial release (MFR), Rolfing®, Soft tissue release (STR), or Structural integration

6. Neuromuscular

7. Decrease pain; improve range of motion; loosen myofascial components

8. Any of the following: Myotherapy, NeuroKinetic Therapy®, Neuromuscular technique (NMT), Positional release therapy (PRT), Proprioceptive neuromuscular facilitation (PNF), Strain-counterstrain, Tender point, or Trigger point

9. Edema uptake, lymph flow, and other lymphatic processes

10. Movement therapies

11. Any of the following: general relaxation and body awareness; neuromuscular reeducation; or release holding patterns (emotional or physical)

12. The use of light or deep pressure to stimulate defined energy zones, dermatomes, or points

13. Any of the following: Amma therapy, Bindegewebsmassage/connective tissue massage (CTM), Reflexology, Shiatsu, or Therapeutic Touch®

14. Energy techniques

15. Any of the following: prana, qi, ki, or life force

16. Any of the following: Chakra balancing, Polarity therapy, Qigong, Reiki®, Touch for Health (TFH), or Therapeutic Touch®

EXERCISE 10 Creating a Body Systems Table

Remember, your answers do not need to be exactly the same as the ones offered here.

1. Protective outer covering; sensory organ; regulation of body temperature

2. Bone, cartilage, and joints

3. Bone landmarks for postural assessment; structural effects on the joint receptors and connective tissues

4. Skeletal muscle and tendon

5. Maintain posture; create movement; generation of heat

6. Brain, spinal cord, nerves, special and general sensory receptors

7. Mediates benefits and physiologic effects of manual therapy

8. Hypothalamus, pituitary, thyroid, parathyroids, thymus, adrenals, pancreas, gonads

9. Benefits such as stress reduction, improved mental focus, and restorative sleep involve changes in endocrine function

10. Transportation of nutrients, wastes, and hormones

11. Manual therapies can improve local blood flow and decrease blood pressure

12. Tonsils, thymus, spleen, white blood cells, lymph nodes, and vessels

13. Fluid and protein return; resistance to disease

14. Regulation and exchange of oxygen and carbon dioxide; vocalization

15. Manual therapies can improve the efficiency and ease of breathing

16. Mouth, salivary glands, esophagus, stomach, small and large intestines, anus, liver, gallbladder, pancreas

17. Breakdown of food; absorption of nutrients; elimination of solid waste

18. Kidneys, ureters, bladder, and urethra

19. Female: ovaries, fallopian tubes, uterus, vagina, and vulva; Male: testes, seminal vesicles, vas deferens, prostate, penis

20. Manual therapies can impact fertility and the reproductive cycle. They can also be used to support people during pregnancy, labor, and childbirth.

EXERCISE 11 Body Systems Anatomy Mind Map

Integumentary: skin, glands, hair, nails, sensory receptors

Nervous: brain, spinal cord, nerves, special sensory receptors, general sensory receptors

Endocrine: thyroid, thymus, gonads, parathyroids, adrenals, pancreas, pituitary, hypothalamus

Reproductive: vulva, uterus, vagina, penis, prostate, tubes, gonads

Urinary: kidneys, ureters, bladder, urethra

Digestive: pancreas, anus, liver, stomach, intestines, esophagus, mouth, gallbladder

Respiratory: bronchi, lungs, trachea, nose, sinuses

Cardiovascular: blood vessels, heart, blood

Lymphatic/immune: lymph nodes, white blood cells, thymus, tonsils, spleen, lymphatic vessels

Muscular: muscle, tendon

Skeletal: bone, joints, cartilage

EXERCISE 12 Body Systems Physiology Mind Map

Integumentary: protection, covering, sensory, regulation of body temperature

Nervous: coordination, communication, control

Endocrine: coordination, communication, control

Reproductive: reproduction

Urinary: cleanse blood, eliminate waste

Digestive: absorb nutrients, eliminate solid wastes, break down food into useable nutrients

Respiratory: oxygen and carbon dioxide exchange

Cardiovascular: transportation

Lymphatic/immune: resistance to disease, fluid and protein return

Muscular: heat, movement, posture

Skeletal: structure, protection, levers, blood cell production, mineral storage

Answers to Chapter 1 quiz

1. A tissue
2. C organs
3. B stimulus
4. B negative
5. C a dynamic equilibrium between physiologic processes needed to sustain life
6. B kidney
7. C lymphatic
8. A endocrine and digestive
9. D blood vessels; heart
10. C Feldenkrais Method®
11. B myofascial/deep tissue
12. D reflexive/zone therapy
13. D benefits of manual therapy
14. C physiologic effects
15. A releasing holding patterns
16. A stretching muscles
17. B Swedish
18. D shiatsu
19. A enhancing general well-being
20. C lymphatic
21. A helping to balance fluids and blood pH
22. C respiratory
23. D muscular
24. B serving as the site of blood cell production
25. A sensory receptors

Chapter 2

EXERCISE 2 Planes of the Body

1. Frontal or coronal
2. Sagittal or median
3. Transverse or horizontal
4. Frontal or coronal
5. Transverse or horizontal
6. Sagittal or median

EXERCISE 3 Location and Movement Terms Crossword

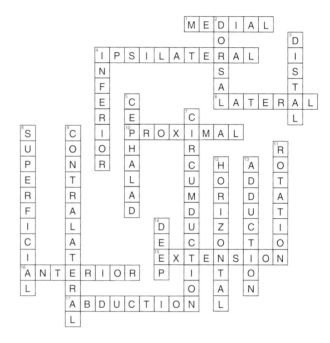

EXERCISE 4 Mix-and-Match Word Parts

1. C unicycle
2. D contradictions
3. H myositis
4. G interosseous membrane
5. A pseudonym
6. I tulipoma
7. J hemisphere
8. B malcontent
9. F retropatellar
10. E antechamber

EXERCISE 5 Body Cavities Color and Label

1. Cranial
2. Spinal
3. Thoracic
4. Abdominopelvic
5. Diaphragm
6. Abdominal
7. Pelvic

EXERCISE 6 Body Regions Matching

1. J fibular
2. D crural
3. G olecranal
4. K coxal
5. B cephalic
6. M thoracic
7. A pedal
8. N sural
9. E temporal
10. F volar
11. H carpal
12. Q occipital
13. T gluteal
14. C inguinal
15. S lumbar
16. I nasal
17. L femoral
18. O axillary
19. P pectoral
20. R popliteal

EXERCISE 7 Body Regions Labeling

1. Frontal
2. Orbital
3. Sternal
4. Pectoral
5. Brachial
6. Antecubital
7. Antebrachial
8. Digital
9. Inguinal
10. Patellar
11. Tarsal
12. Acromial
13. Cervical
14. Scapular
15. Vertebral or spinal
16. Sacral
17. Popliteal
18. Sural
19. Calcaneal
20. Plantar

EXERCISE 8 Pathology Terms Case Report

1. Etiology is infected tonsils.
2. Diagnosis is tonsillitis.
3. Symptoms include headache; feeling tired and generally run-down; a throat that feels scratchy and swollen; painful swallowing; trouble sleeping.
4. Signs include swollen lymph nodes in his neck, a fever of 102°F, and red and pus-marked tonsils causing severe sore throat.
5. Prognosis is for a complete recovery within 2 or 3 days after surgery with a prescription of antibiotics.

EXERCISE 9 Classes of Disease Table

1. Disease caused by a specific pathogen such as a bacteria, virus, fungus, or parasite, which creates a physiologic disruption
2. Examples include the common cold, influenza, tuberculosis, malaria, dysentery, tapeworms, lice, and many more.
3. Environmental
4. Disease caused by exposure to harmful substances in surroundings
5. Hereditary
6. Examples include hemophilia, sickle cell anemia, Down syndrome, polycystic kidney disease, muscular dystrophy, and many more.
7. Disease related to poor nutrition or unhealthy lifestyle
8. Examples include scurvy, anemia, type 2 diabetes, osteoporosis, atherosclerosis, and some types of cancer.
9. Autoimmune
10. A disorder caused by the immune system mistakenly attacking and destroying a part of the body
11. Cancerous
12. Melanoma, leukemia, myeloma, and many others

EXERCISE 10 A&P Terminology Crossword

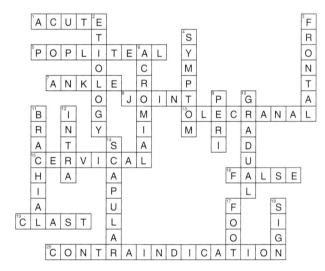

Answers to Chapter 2 quiz

1. B frontal/coronal
2. A sagittal/median
3. D thoracic and abdominopelvic
4. D medial/lateral
5. B closer to the head
6. A contralateral
7. C proximal
8. A cranial
9. D popliteal
10. B axilla
11. A groin
12. C flexion
13. D rotation
14. A infra-
15. C cell
16. C endo-
17. A upper right
18. D elbow
19. A pathogen
20. B environmental
21. C etiology
22. D acute
23. A parasites
24. C contagious
25. B autoimmune

Chapter 3

EXERCISE 1 Chemistry Crossword

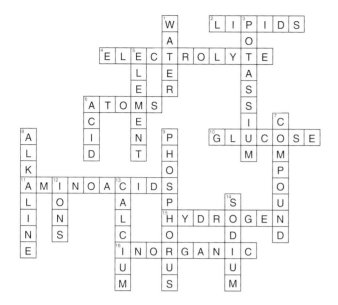

EXERCISE 2 Cellular Components Flow Chart

1. Phospholipid
2. IMPs
3. Receptor proteins
4. Effector proteins
5–7. Channel proteins, transport proteins, linker proteins
8. Cytosol
9. Organic compounds
10. Organelles
11–16. Mitochondria, lysosomes, Golgi apparatus, vesicle, cytoskeleton, centrosome
17. Endoplasmic reticulum
18. Ribosomes
19. Genetic blueprint
20. Nuclear envelope
21. Nucleolus
22. DNA
23. Genes

EXERCISE 3 Cell Diagram

1. Ribosome
2. Rough ER
3. Smooth ER
4. Cytoskeleton
5. Centrosome
6. Protein
7. Lysosome
8. Mitochondrion
9. Plasma or cell membrane
10. Cytosol
11. Golgi apparatus
12. Nuclear envelope
13. Nucleolus
14. Nucleus

EXERCISE 4 A Cell Analogy

1. Plasma membrane
2. Nucleus
3. DNA
4. Mitochondria
5. Ribosomes
6. Golgi apparatus
7. Lysosomes
8. Endoplasmic reticulum
9. Rough
10. Smooth

EXERCISE 5 Cellular Transport

1. Intracellular fluid
2. Extracellular fluid
3. Interstitial fluid
4. Passive
5. Active
A. Diffusion
B. Osmosis
C. Phagocytosis

EXERCISE 6 Cellular Processes Matching

1. D metabolism
2. I catabolism
3. F anabolism
4. L protein synthesis
5. A glycogen
6. N mitosis
7. B cytokinesis
8. H meiosis
9. O differentiation
10. C stem cell
11. K embryonic layer
12. M filtration
13. G cell division
14. E phagocytosis
15. J exocytosis

Answers to Chapter 3 quiz

1. A cytoplasm
2. C water
3. C stratified squamous
4. D adipose
5. B element
6. A acidic
7. B proteins
8. B monitor the internal and external environment of the cell
9. C endoplasmic reticulum
10. C mitochondria
11. A ribosomes
12. B filtration
13. C osmosis
14. D sodium pump
15. B mitosis
16. A differentiation
17. D muscle, epithelial, connective, nerve
18. A smooth and involuntary
19. A neuroglia
20. C epithelial
21. C striated and involuntary
22. A direct the responses of the cell according to information from receptor proteins
23. D any process used to break down nutrients or molecules
24. C multipotent
25. B neuronal

Answer Key   207

Chapter 4

EXERCISE 1 Terminology Crossword

	¹H		²A			³S			⁴M						
	Y		P		⁵M	U	S	C	L	E		⁶S	E	B	U	M	⁷M

(Crossword answers)

Across/Down filled letters:
- H Y P O D E R M I S
- A P O C R I N E
- S U D O R I F E R O U S
- M U S C L E
- M E L A N O V I S C A R I N E
- S E B U M
- M E L A N O M A
- N O C I C E P T O R
- K E R A T I N
- E C C R I N E
- R E T I C U L A R
- S T R A T A
- S A L L
- M U C U S
- T I L
- V I S C E R A L
- D E R M I S
- E X T E N S I B L E

EXERCISE 2 Membranes Organizational Chart

1. A broad flat sheet of at least two layers of tissue
2. Connective tissue membranes
3. Epithelial membranes
4. Synovial membranes; structure—thick fibrous connective tissue layer with a thin internal layer of simple epithelium; function—line synovial joint cavities and secrete synovial fluid; examples—knee, ankle, elbow, shoulder, hip
5. Mucous membranes; structure—simple columnar epithelium attached to a thin basement membrane; function—line cavities with openings to the external environment and secrete mucus; examples—lining respiratory, digestive, urinary, and reproductive tracts
6. Serous membranes; structure—thin simple epithelial layer attached to a basement membrane, folds into two layers, called parietal and visceral layers; function—parietal layer lines cavities without openings to the external environment and visceral layer covers internal organs; examples—pleura in the thoracic cavity, peritoneum of the abdominopelvic cavity
7. Cutaneous membrane; structure—epidermis and dermis; function—protection, temperature regulation, excretion, absorption, general sensory organ, and synthesis of vitamin D; example—the skin

EXERCISE 3 Functional Mnemonic

The mnemonic will differ; however, here is a summary of the functions:

Protection—Serves as a physical barrier to pathogens and contaminants.

Temperature regulation—Sweat helps to cool us and the hypodermis insulates to help us retain body heat.

Excretion—Sweating eliminates trace amounts of metabolic waste products.

Absorption—Oils, herbal extracts, or medications can be absorbed through the layers of the cutaneous membrane.

General sensory organ—Numerous cutaneous receptors collect information about what is happening to the surface of the body.

Synthesis of vitamin D—Ultraviolet light absorbed by the skin stimulates the synthesis of vitamin D.

EXERCISE 4 Skin Diagram

1. Epidermis
2. Dermis
3. Hypodermis
4. Hair shaft
5. Hair root
6. Sebaceous gland
7. Arrector pili muscle
8. Hair follicle
9. Apocrine sweat gland
10. Blood vessels
11. Fat /adipose tissue
12. Sensory receptors
13. Nerve
14. Pore
15. Eccrine sweat gland

EXERCISE 6 Matching Structures and Functions

1. E hair follicle
2. I fingernail
3. D arrector pili
4. L sebaceous gland
5. C sudoriferous gland
6. H eccrine gland
7. M apocrine gland
8. B nociceptor
9. K Merkel disc
10. F Meissner's corpuscle
11. N Pacinian corpuscle
12. G Ruffini's corpuscle
13. J hair root plexus
14. O sebum
15. A epidermis

EXERCISE 7 Pathology Mind Map

1–4. Fungal infections, Bacterial infections, Viral infections, Parasitic infections

5–9. Acne, Eczema, Hives, Psoriasis, Vitiligo

Answers to Chapter 4 quiz

1. B two or more layers of tissue that generally serve as coverings or linings to other structures
2. C synovial, mucous, cutaneous, serous
3. C serve as large sensory organ; produce vitamin D
4. D visceral pleura
5. A free nerve endings; Merkel discs
6. C cutaneous
7. B epidermis
8. A germinating
9. C toughen and waterproof the skin

10. D melanin
11. B composed of numerous layers of epithelial cells
12. B dermis
13. D papillary
14. A insulation and energy storage
15. B sebaceous
16. C apocrine
17. D free nerve endings
18. C eccrine glands
19. C vibration
20. A dermatome
21. D vitiligo
22. C tinea pedis
23. A shingles
24. B scabies and lice
25. B MRSA

Chapter 5

EXERCISE 1 Bony Terms Crossword

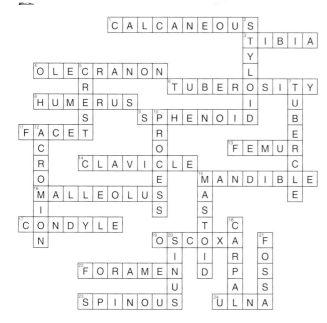

EXERCISE 3 Label the Skeleton

1. Cranium
2. Facial bones
3. Hyoid
4. Clavicle
5. Scapula
6. Sternum
7. Ribs (costal bones)
8. Humerus
9. Radius
10. Ulna
11. Carpals
12. Metacarpals
13. Phalanges
14. Femur
15. Patella
16. Tibia
17. Fibula
18. Tarsals
19. Metatarsals
20. Phalanges
21. Ilium
22. Pubis
23. Ischium
24. Coxal bone
25. Vertebra
26. Sacrum
27. Coccyx

EXERCISE 4 Draw Me a Bone

Short bones—carpals and tarsals
Long bones—humerus, radius, ulna, femur, tibia, fibula
Flat bones—cranial bones, mandible, ribs, sternum
Irregular bones—scapula, vertebra, pelvic bones

EXERCISE 5 Parts of a Long Bone

Matching portion:

1. C epiphysis
2. I articular cartilage
3. F red bone marrow
4. A epiphyseal line
5. K spongy bone
6. E metaphysis
7. J diaphysis
8. B periosteum
9. L endosteum
10. H medullary cavity
11. D yellow bone marrow
12. G compact bone

Labeling portion:

1. Epiphysis
2. Metaphysis
3. Diaphysis
4. Articular cartilage (hyaline)
5. Red marrow
6. Epiphyseal line
7. Spongy bone
8. Endosteum
9. Medullary cavity
10. Yellow marrow
11. Compact bone
12. Periosteum

EXERCISE 6 Build a Long Bone

1. Diaphysis
2. Medullary cavity
3. Yellow bone marrow
4. Epiphyses
5. Red bone marrow
6. Articular cartilage
7. Periosteum

EXERCISE 7 Skeletal Landmarks Labeling

1. H iliac crest
2. N lateral malleolus
3. K greater trochanter
4. A occipital bone
5. F olecranon process
6. O calcaneus
7. L patella
8. E inferior angle of scapula
9. C mastoid process
10. D acromion process
11. B mandible
12. M tibial tuberosity
13. G head of radius
14. I ASIS
15. J ischial tuberosity
16. P glenoid fossa
17. S spinous process
18. T lateral humeral epicondyle
19. Q xiphoid process
20. R crest of tibia

Answer Key 209

EXERCISE 8 Label a Synovial Joint

1. Synovial membrane
2. Anterior cruciate ligament
3. Fibrous joint capsule
4. Menisci
5. Synovial fluid
6. Bursa
7. Patella
8. Fat pad
9. Articular cartilage
10. Patellar ligament

EXERCISE 9 Diarthrotic Joint Movements

1. Pivot
2. Rotation
3. Ball-and-socket
4. Flexion, extension, ABduction, adduction, rotation, circumduction
5. Pivot
6. Rotation
7. Hinge
8. Flexion, extension
9. Condyloid
10. Flexion, extension, ABduction, adduction
11. Saddle
12. Flexion, extension, ABduction, adduction
13. Condyloid
14. Flexion, extension, ABduction, adduction
15. Hinge
16. Flexion, extension
17. Ball-and-socket
18. Flexion, extension, ABduction, adduction, rotation, circumduction
19. Hinge
20. Flexion, extension
21. Hinge
22. Dorsiflexion, plantar flexion
23. Gliding
24. Sliding, shifting for inversion, eversion

EXERCISE 10 Joint Crossword

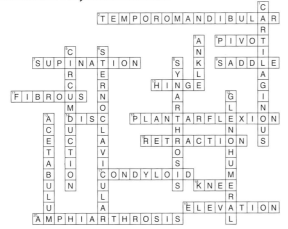

Answers to Chapter 5 quiz

1. C protecting vital organs; storing calcium and minerals
2. D flat; irregular
3. A cartilaginous
4. D ball-and-socket
5. B hinge
6. B synarthrosis
7. C sacrum
8. A scapula
9. B lacrimal
10. C clavicle
11. B phalanges
12. A epiphyses
13. A compact
14. D medullary
15. B epiphysis
16. B hyaline cartilage
17. C fibula
18. C 7
19. A 7
20. D manubrium
21. C pubic symphysis
22. A metacarpophalangeal
23. C acromion
24. D cortical
25. A haversian

Chapter 6

EXERCISE 1 Muscle Terminology Crossword

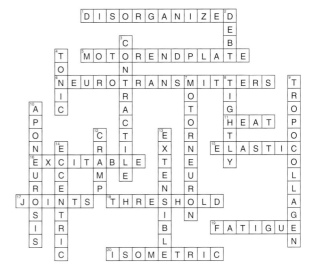

EXERCISE 2 Major Parts of a Skeletal Muscle

1. Bone
2. Tendon
3. Tenoperiosteal junction
4. Musculotendinous junction
5. Epimysium
6. Perimysium
7. Fascicle
8. Endomysium
9. Fiber (muscle cell)
10. Sarcolemma

EXERCISE 3 Comparing Fascia and Tendons

There are many possible answers for this exercise. Some examples include the ones listed in the diagram below:

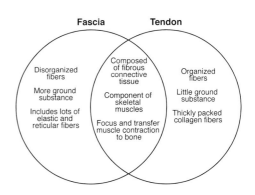

210   Answer Key

EXERCISE 4 Skeletal Muscle Fiber Organization

1. F muscle fiber
2. D myofibrils
3. J mitochondrion
4. A sarcoplasmic reticulum
5. K sarcolemma
6. E myofilaments
7. I myosin
8. B actin
9. L Z line
10. H A band
11. C I band
12. G sarcomere

EXERCISE 5 Muscle Microanatomy

1. Sarcomere
2. Myosin
3. Actin
4. Z lines
5. A band
6. I bands
7. Myofilaments (actin and myosin)
8. Myofibril
9. Mitochondrion
10. Nucleus
11. Sarcoplasmic reticulum
12. Sarcolemma

EXERCISE 6 Skeletal Muscle Contraction

1. Sliding filament mechanism
2. Sarcomeres
3. Motor unit
4. Motor neuron
5. Fibers
6. Neuromuscular junction
7. Neurotransmitters
8. Motor neuron
9. Motor end plates
10. Threshold stimulus
11. All-or-none response
12. Threshold
13. All
14. None
15–16. Graded response; motor unit recruitment
17. Calcium
18. Sarcoplasmic reticulum
19. Actin filaments
20. Myosin heads
21. Pull the two myofilaments across one another
22. Myosin heads
23. Continued sliding of the filaments across one another
24. Calcium
25. Sarcoplasmic reticulum

EXERCISE 7 Picturing Energy for Muscle Contraction

1. Creatine phosphate
2. ADP
3. ATP
4. Creatine
5. Glucose
6. 2 ATP
7. Lactic acid
8. Anaerobic
9. Pyruvic acid
10. Krebs
11. 30–32 ATP
12–14. H_2O, CO_2, and heat
15. Aerobic

EXERCISE 8 Organizing Methods of ATP Production

1. Direct phosphorylation
2. ATP + creatine
3. Glucose is converted into pyruvic acid to release ATP.
4. No, anaerobic process
5. Aerobic cellular metabolism or Krebs cycle
6. Pyruvic acid is converted into H_2O and CO_2, releasing heat and providing ATP (can also convert fatty acids and amino acids into energy).
7. H_2O, CO_2, and heat plus lots of ATP

EXERCISE 9 Types of Fiber Arrangements

Specific muscle examples may differ. Check with your instructor.

1. Infrahyoids, rectus abdominis
2. Fusiform
3. Circular
4. Pectoralis major, latissimus dorsi
5. Extensor digitorum longus, fibularis longus
6. Bipennate
7. Multipennate

EXERCISE 10 Muscle Assignments

Agonist—This muscle is generally the largest and the strongest or has the best angle of pull across a joint to its attachment point; the prime mover.

Antagonist—A muscle that opposes the agonist.

Synergist—A muscle that helps or assists the prime mover.

Stabilizer—A muscle that stabilizes the prime mover's bone of origin to make the movement created by the agonist more efficient.

Answers for the table may differ. If you have questions or your answer does not appear below, check with your fellow classmates or instructor.

1. Biceps femoris, semimembranosus, or semitendinosus
2. Vastus medialis, vastus intermedius, or vastus lateralis
3. Biceps femoris
4. Rectus femoris, vastus medialis, vastus intermedius, or vastus lateralis
5. Latissimus dorsi or posterior deltoid
6. Pectoralis major, coracobrachialis, or anterior deltoid
7. Latissimus dorsi, teres major, or posterior deltoid
8. Depending on specific answer to No. 6, could be pectoralis major, coracobrachialis, anterior deltoid, or biceps brachii
9. Deltoid

Answers for Exercise 10 continued on next page.

EXERCISE 10 Muscle Assignments, continued

10. Pectoralis major, coracobrachialis, latissimus dorsi, or teres major

11. Deltoid

12. Coracobrachialis, latissimus dorsi, or teres major

13. Infraspinatus, teres minor, posterior deltoid

14. Subscapularis, pectoralis major, latissimus dorsi, teres major, or anterior deltoid

15. Teres minor, posterior deltoid

EXERCISE 11 Naming Muscles

While your specific muscle examples may differ, the naming themes and some examples include

Shape—Deltoid, rhomboids, quadratus lumborum

Function—Supinator, pronator teres, extensor digitorum, flexor digitorum, flexor hallucis

Fiber direction—Rectus abdominis, external obliques, internal obliques, transverse abdominis

General location—Tibialis anterior, tibialis posterior, brachialis

Origin or insertion—Sternocleidomastoid, coracobrachialis, palmaris longus, brachoradialis

Number of origins—Biceps brachii, triceps brachii, biceps femoris

EXERCISE 12 Locating Major Muscles

Anterior view:

1. Temporalis
2. Orbicularis oculi
3. Masseter
4. Sternocleidomastoid
5. Trapezius
6. Deltoid
7. Pectoralis major
8. Serratus anterior
9. Biceps brachii
10. Brachialis
11. Brachioradialis
12. Flexor carpi radialis
13. Palmaris longus
14. Fibularis longus
15. Tibialis anterior
16. Vastus medialis

17. Rectus femoris
18. Vastus lateralis
19. Gracilis
20. Sartorius
21. Adductor longus
22. Pectineus
23. Iliopsoas
24. Tensor fasciae latae
25. Extensor digitorum superficialis
26. Extensor carpi radialis
27. External obliques
28. Rectus abdominis
29. Internal obliques
30. Orbicularis oris
31. Zygomaticus
32. Frontalis

Posterior view:

1. Temporalis
2. Masseter
3. Infraspinatus
4. Teres minor
5. Teres major
6. Latissimus dorsi
7. External obliques
8. Flexor carpi ulnaris
9. Extensor carpi ulnaris
10. Gluteus medius
11. Gluteus maximus
12. Adductor magnus
13. Iliotibial tract or band
14. Gracilis
15. Gastrocnemius
16. Fibularis longus

17. Soleus
18. Soleus
19. Semimembranosus
20. Semitendinosus
21. Biceps femoris
22. Flexor carpi ulnaris
23. Extensor carpi ulnaris
24. Extensor digitorum superficialis
25. Extensor carpi radialis
26. Brachioradialis
27. Triceps brachii
28. Deltoid
29. Trapezius
30. Occipitalis

Answers to Chapter 6 quiz

1. B create movement, help stabilize joints, maintain posture, and generate heat
2. C extensible; elastic
3. C latissimus dorsi and iliocostalis
4. A All fibers in a motor unit must contract fully when sufficient stimulus is delivered.
5. A calcium
6. D sarcomere
7. C fascicle
8. D lots of ground substance that keeps fibers widely spaced
9. B multiple muscle fibers
10. A increasing or decreasing the number of motor units stimulated

11. C threshold stimulus
12. D direct phosphorylation (ATP-CP)
13. B anaerobic cellular metabolism
14. B tonic
15. D isometric
16. D parallel
17. A oppose the primary movement
18. C origin
19. C muscle tone
20. A concentric isotomic
21. C passive
22. B knee extension
23. B brachialis
24. D teres minor
25. C gracilis

Chapter 7

EXERCISE 1 Nervous System Crossword

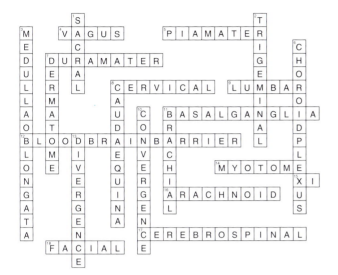

EXERCISE 2 Functional Organization of the Nervous System

1. Central nervous system
2. Peripheral nervous system
3. Spinal cord
4–7. Cerebrum, Diencephalon, Brain stem, Cerebellum
8. Somatic division
9. Sympathetic division
10. Parasympathetic division

EXERCISE 3 Neuroglia Mind Map

1. Microglia
2. Satellite cells
3. Oligodendrocytes
4–5. Maintenance of chemical environment for impulse conduction, scar tissue formation
6. Form CSF
7. Make and maintain myelin in the PNS

Astrocytes and Ependymal cells

Schwann cells

EXERCISE 4 Matching Neuron Parts

1. D axon
2. J axon hillock
3. A axon terminal
4. N myelin
5. G cell body
6. E dendrites
7. L nucleus
8. B sensory neuron
9. O interneuron
10. C motor neuron
11. M unipolar
12. K bipolar
13. H multipolar
14. F neurilemma
15. I synaptic bulb

EXERCISE 5 Neurons and Their Parts

1. Dendrites
2. Cell body
3. Nucleus
4. Axon hillock
5. Axon
6. Myelin
7. Axon terminal with synaptic bulb
8. Unipolar
9. Bipolar
10. Multipolar

EXERCISE 6 Structure of a Nerve

13 pairs of cranial nerves

31 pairs of spinal nerves

Diagram:

1. Epineurium
2. Fascicle
3. Perineurium
4. Nerve fibers (axons)
5. Endoneurium
6. Schwann cells
7. Myelin
8. Axon
9. Artery and vein (blood vessels)

EXERCISE 8 Diagram a Reflex Arc

1. Outcome or response
2. Stimulus
3. Two-neuron
4. Three-neuron
5. Spinal cord
6. Sensory receptors (stretch receptors in skeletal muscle)
7. Sensory neuron
8. Sensory receptors (pain receptors in skin)
9. Sensory neuron
10. Synapse
11. Interneuron
12. Motor neuron
13. Skeletal muscle effector or quadriceps
14. Skeletal muscle effector or biceps

Answer Key   213

EXERCISE 9 Sensory Receptors Table

1. Photoreceptors
2. Retina of the eye
3. Tissue damage (pain)
4. Skin, joint capsules, fascia, periosteum, blood vessel walls
5. Proprioceptors
6. Movement, muscle tension, and length of muscles
7. Touch, pressure, and movement stimulus such as stretch, compression, and torsion
8. Skin, hollow organs, cochlea, and bony labyrinth of the ear
9. Chemoreceptors
10. Nose, tongue, and blood vessels
11. Temperature changes
12. Skin

EXERCISE 10 Meninges Diagram

1. Dura mater
2. Arachnoid mater
3. Subarachnoid space
4. Arachnoid villus
5. Pia mater

EXERCISE 11 Nervous Terminology: Reviewing Synonyms

1. Afferent
2. Motor
3. Ascending, sensory, afferent, posterior, or dorsal tracts
4. Descending, motor, efferent, anterior, or ventral tracts
5. Dorsal, sensory, afferent, or posterior root
6. Ventral, motor, efferent, or anterior root

EXERCISE 12 Spinal Cord Gray Matter Organization

1. Posterior
2. Lateral
3. Anterior
4. Somatic sensory
5. Visceral sensory
6. Visceral motor
7. Somatic motor

EXERCISE 13 Matching Brain Parts and Their Functions

1. Cerebrum, G
2. Corpus callosum, C
3. Thalamus, A
4. Hypothalamus, F
5. Pituitary gland, D
6. Pineal gland, K
7. Midbrain, I
8. Pons, H
9. Medulla oblongata, B
10. Reticular formation, J
11. Cerebellum, E

EXERCISE 14 Cerebral Structures

Fill in the blank:

1. Gyri (singular gyrus)
2. Fissures
3. Hemispheres
4. Sulci (singular sulcus)
5. Lobes

Diagram labels:

1. Longitudinal fissure
2. Transverse fissure
3. Right cerebral hemisphere
4. Left cerebral hemisphere
5. Central sulcus
6. Lateral sulcus
7. Frontal lobe
8. Parietal lobe
9. Temporal lobe
10. Occipital lobe

EXERCISE 15 Pathways of the Nervous System

Neurons and tracts:

A sensory neurons
B somatic motor neurons
D sympathetic motor neurons
C parasympathetic motor neurons
F ascending tracts
E descending tracts

Brain and cord:

5 spinal cord
6 cauda equina
1 cerebrum
2 diencephalon
3 brain stem
4 cerebellum

EXERCISE 16 Comparing Somatic and Autonomic Motor Pathways

There are many possible answers for this exercise. Some examples include the following:

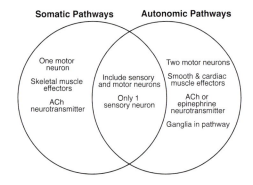

214   Answer Key

EXERCISE 17 ANS Features

1. Fight-or-flight
2. Feed-and-breed
3. Thoracolumbar
4. Craniosacral
5. 2
6. 2
7. Paravertebral chain
8. In or near effector
9. Widespread
10. Targeted
11. Norepinephrine
12. Acetylcholine

Answers to Chapter 7 quiz

1. C integration; motor
2. B associative, sensory, motor
3. D oligodendrocytes
4. A brain stem, cerebrum, diencephalon, cerebellum
5. B trigeminal
6. C C-7 and T-1
7. A brachial
8. C femoral and lateral femoral cutaneous
9. D cerebellum
10. B action potential
11. A neurotransmitters
12. C divergence
13. D biceps femoris
14. A taste and smell
15. D two motor neurons
16. B rapid lengthening
17. D ascending and dorsal tracts
18. B arachnoid
19. A act as the medium for nutrient waste exchange
20. C loss of movement and/or muscle strength
21. D medulla oblongata
22. B thalamus
23. C junction between the two cerebral hemispheres
24. D limbic system
25. B hypothalamus

Chapter 8

EXERCISE 1 Neuromuscular and Myofascial Terminology Crossword

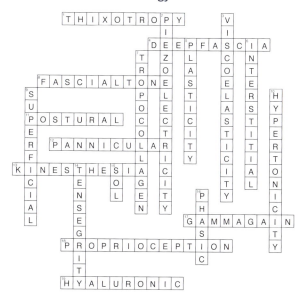

EXERCISE 2 Neuromuscular Reflexes Table

1. A
2. G
3. C
4. D
5. E
6. B
7. F

EXERCISE 3 Neuronal Loops

1. Lengthening
2. Contraction
3. Stretch reflex
4. Alpha sensory
5. Alpha motor
6. Extrafusal
7. Stretch reflex
8. Control and coordinate voluntary movement
9. Gamma loop
10. Gamma sensory stretching
11. Gamma motor
12. Intrafusal
13. Sensitivity
14. Length; tension
15. Tension
16. Sensitivity
17. Gamma gain or loading

EXERCISE 4 Trigger Versus Tender Points

1. TeP
2. B
3. TeP
4. TP
5. TP
6. TP
7. TP
8. TeP
9. TeP
10. TP
11. TeP
12. TeP

EXERCISE 5 Tensegrity

1. Tension
2. Integrity
3. Compression
4. Tension
5. Upright posture

There are many possible examples, especially because all homeostatic mechanisms are basically functional tensegrity systems. For example, pH is balancing acidity vs. alkalinity, and hormones balance too much vs. too little glucose in the blood.

EXERCISE 6 Fascial Layers and Planes

1. Lumbosacral aponeurosis

2–4. Blood vessels, nerves, organs

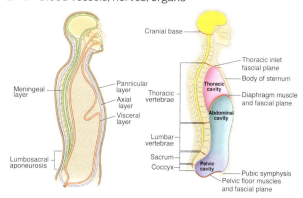

EXERCISE 7 Mechanical Properties of Fascia

1. The ability of tissues to extend and rebound rather than stretch and recoil

2. The ability to vacillate between a more viscous (gel) state and more liquid (sol) state in response to temperature or movement

3. The ability to produce a small electrical charge in response to mechanical pressure

4. Slow, steady pace; gradual application of superficial to deep pressure to assist in warming; constant movement of tissue with hands (instrument) to maintain warming and increase soluble change; increased duration to fully effect change

5. Sustained, moderate pressure and movement to affect fascial components

EXERCISE 8 Fascial Receptors

1. P
2. R
3. GO
4. IMF
5. P
6. IMF
7. R
8. P
9. IMF
10. GO

EXERCISE 9 Concepts in Posture, Balance, and Coordinated Movement

1. G muscle tone
2. B phasic muscle
3. A muscle recruitment
4. F motor tone
5. H neurofascial loops
6. E motor unit recruitment
7. D fascial tone
8. C postural muscle

Answers to Chapter 8 quiz

1. D viscoelasticity, piezoelectricity, and thixotropic
2. A the pattern of coactivation between muscle groups needed to create coordinated movement
3. C reciprocal inhibition
4. B gamma gain
5. A alpha
6. D Rolfing
7. C active muscle contraction
8. C a shortened position
9. A a common pattern of pain with pressure and a palpable nodule within a taut band of tissue
10. D triceps brachii

11. A The presence of calcium outside of the sarcoplasmic reticulum causes actin and myosin bonding.

12. D tensegrity

13. B provide some stability to the torso by strapping the soft anterior structures to the spine

14. D structurally divide both anterior and posterior cavities and support blood vessels and nerves

15. D local muscle spasm indicating a sensitized muscle spindle

16. B visceral

17. C superficial back line

18. A thoracic inlet

19. A viscoelasticity

20. C Ruffini's receptors

21. D interstitial myofascial

22. B autonomic nervous system

23. B motor tone

24. C kinesthesia

25. D Type I fibers

Chapter 9

EXERCISE 1 Endocrine System Crossword

EXERCISE 2 Locating Endocrine Glands

1. Hypothalamus
2. Pituitary
3. Pineal
4. Thyroid
5. Parathyroids
6. Thymus
7. Adrenal
8. Pancreas
9. Gonads

EXERCISE 3 Comparing the Communication Systems

1. No
2. Yes
3. Slow
4. Immediate
5. Long-term change like growth and maturation
6. Short-term, instantaneous changes like movement, breathing, and heart rate
7. Pituitary (endocrine gland connected to the hypothalamus)
8. Hypothalamus (brain region connected to the pituitary)
9. Hormones through the bloodstream
10. Nerve impulses along neurons

EXERCISE 4 Mechanisms of Hormone Action

1. Water-soluble
2. Plasma membrane
3. G-protein
4. Cyclic AMP (cAMP)
5. Physiologic change or cellular response
6. Second-messenger mechanism
7. Lipid-soluble
8. Plasma (or cell) membrane
9. Cytoplasm
10. Nuclear membrane
11. DNA
12. mRNA
13. Protein

EXERCISE 5 Stimulating and Regulating Hormone Activity

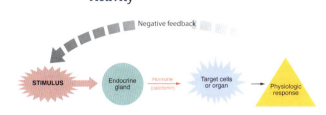

1. Hormonal stimulus—Hypothalamus stimulates the anterior pituitary; anterior pituitary stimulates the gonads, thyroid, and a portion of the adrenal cortex.
2. Changes in blood concentrations—Calcitonin release from the thyroid gland; PTH from the parathyroid; glucagon and insulin from the pancreas.
3. Neurologic stimulus—Hypothalamus and posterior pituitary, and the sympathetic stimulation of the adrenal glands.

EXERCISE 6 Glands and Their Hormones

Pineal—melatonin

Anterior pituitary—TSH, ACTH, FSH, LH, prolactin, and GH

Posterior pituitary—ADH and oxytocin

Thyroid—T_3, T_4, and calcitonin

Parathyroids—PTH

Thymus—thymosin

Adrenals—mineralocorticoids (aldosterone), glucocorticoids (cortisol), and androgens (DHEA) from the cortex; catecholamines (adrenaline and noradrenaline) from the medulla

Pancreas—insulin and glucagon

Ovaries—estrogens and progesterone

Testes—testosterone (androgens)

EXERCISE 7 Matching Hormones and Physiologic Responses

1. R   ACTH
2. G   glucagon
3. J   PTH
4. E   testosterone
5. I   thymosin
6. Q   LH
7. B   cortisol
8. O   GH
9. P   prolactin
10. C   adrenaline
11. N   oxytocin
12. D   estrogen
13. K   calcitonin
14. F   progesterone
15. L   thyroxine
16. H   insulin
17. A   aldosterone
18. M   melatonin

EXERCISE 8 Diagramming Stress

1. Hypothalamus
2. Alarm Response
3. Resistance Reaction
4. Sympathetic nervous system
5. Endocrine system (pituitary)
6. Release of catecholamines from the medulla, which support and prolong
7. ↑ HR, ↑ breathing, dilate bronchioles, dilate pupils, changes in blood flow patterns, ↓ digestion, etc.
8. Adrenals
9. Liver
10. Thyroid
11. Aldosterone ↑ sodium retention to ↑ BP; Cortisol to ↓ inflammatory response
12. Exhaustion

Answers to Chapter 9 quiz

1. C follicle-stimulating (FSH); luteinizing (LH)
2. D homeostatic balance of the blood
3. C water-soluble
4. A second-messenger mechanism
5. B oxytocin
6. C adenohypophysis; neurohypophysis
7. C they do not have a specific duct for the secretions
8. C neurologic stimulus of a specific gland
9. B ACTH
10. D T_3
11. C hypothalamus
12. B parathyroid hormone
13. A calcitriol
14. C adrenals
15. A stimulate or inhibit release of anterior pituitary hormones
16. B increase sodium retention
17. D cortisol
18. B beta
19. C decrease blood glucose levels
20. D pancreas
21. A growth hormone
22. B aldosterone
23. B adrenal cortex
24. A increased blood volume and blood pressure
25. C cortisol

Chapter 10

EXERCISE 1 Cardiovascular Crossword

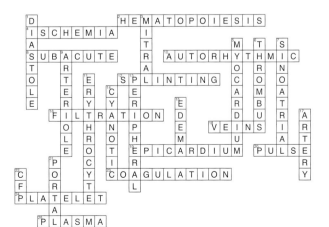

EXERCISE 2 Matching Blood Components

1. C water
2. I hemoglobin
3. E erythrocytes
4. H thrombocytes
5. B globulins
6. F leukocytes
7. A albumins
8. J neutrophils
9. D fibrinogen
10. G lymphocytes

EXERCISE 3 Blood Vessel Structure

1. Artery
2. Arteriole
3. Capillary
4. Venule
5. Vein
A. Inner layer (tunica interna)
A₁. Endothelium
A₂. Basement membrane
B. Middle layer (tunica media)
B₁. Elastic fiber
B₂. Smooth muscle
C. Outer layer (tunica externa)
D. Valve

EXERCISE 5 Primary Arteries of the Body

1. I (pulse point)
2. E (pulse point)
3. R (pulse point)
4. N
5. H (pulse point)
6. O (pulse point)
7. M
8. A (pulse point)
9. B
10. G
11. L
12. J (pulse point)
13. P (pulse point)
14. C
15. F (pulse point)
16. K
17. D
18. Q (pulse point)

EXERCISE 6 Primary Veins of the Body

1. R
2. N
3. A
4. O
5. G
6. H
7. P
8. T
9. M
10. D
11. I
12. J
13. C
14. L
15. K
16. B
17. F
18. E
19. Q
20. S

EXERCISE 7 The Layers of the Heart

1. Fibrous pericardium
2. Serous pericardium (parietal layer)
3. Pericardial cavity or space
4. Serous pericardium (visceral layer) or epicardium (actual heart wall)
5. Myocardium (actual heart wall)
6. Endocardium (actual heart wall)

EXERCISE 8 Blood Flow through the Heart

Diagram structures:

1. Ascending aorta
2. Superior vena cava
3. Right atrium
4. Fossa ovalis
5. Coronary sinus
6. Inferior vena cava
7. Tricuspid valve
8. Right ventricle
9. Intraventricular septum
10. Left ventricle
11. Bicuspid or mitral valve
12. Aortic valve
13. Left atrium
14. Pulmonary veins
15. Pulmonary valve
16. Pulmonary trunk (arterial)

Blood flow:

1—Right atrium
8—Left atrium
3—Right ventricle
10—Left ventricle
9—Bicuspid valve
2—Tricuspid valve
11—Aortic valve
4—Pulmonary valve
12—Aorta
14—Vena cavae
7—Pulmonary veins
5—Pulmonary arteries
13—Systemic capillaries
6—Lung capillaries

EXERCISE 9 The Conduction System of the Heart

Matching:

1. D atrioventricular node
2. E Purkinje fibers
3. B AV bundle
4. C bundle branches
5. A sinoatrial node

Diagram:

1. SA node initiates signal.
2. Signal passes through atria, stimulating contraction.
3. Signal is delayed at AV node.
4. AV bundle passes signal through to the interventricular septum.
5. Bundle branches pass signal down to the apex.
6. Purkinje fibers carry signal through the ventricles, creating a wringing action.

EXERCISE 10 The Cardiac Cycle

Relaxation Phase

Atria are relaxed

Ventricles are relaxed

Semilunar valves are closed

AV valves are open

Blood flows from atria to ventricles

Atrial Systole

Atria are contracted

Ventricles are relaxed

Semilunar valves are closed

AV valves are open

Blood flows from atria to ventricles

Ventricular Systole

Atria are relaxed

Ventricles are contracted

Semilunar valves are open

AV valves are closed

Blood flows from ventricles to great vessels

EXERCISE 11 Cardiovascular Circulation

Right side of heart is blue, while left side is red

1. Pulmonary circuit
2. Systemic circuit
3. Aorta
4. Systemic arterioles
5. Systemic capillaries
6. Systemic venules
7. Superior and inferior vena cavae
8. Pulmonary arteries
9. Pulmonary arterioles
10. Pulmonary capillaries
11. Pulmonary venules
12. Pulmonary veins

EXERCISE 12 Blood Flow

1. Ventricular contraction
2. Arterial recoil
3. Volume
4. Rate
5. Skeletal muscle contractions
6. Valves
7. Respiratory pump

EXERCISE 13 Blood Pressure Regulation

1. Hydrostatic force generated by blood against the vascular wall
2. Systolic
3. Ventricular contraction
4. Diastolic
5. Ventricle relaxes
6. ↑
7. ↑
8. ↓
9. ↑
10. ↓
11. ↑
12. ↓

EXERCISE 14 Capillary Flow

1. Diffusion
2. Glucose, oxygen, carbon dioxide
3. Starling forces
4. Capillary fluid
5. Interstitial fluid
6. Plasma oncotic
7. Protein
8. Interstitial oncotic
9. Filtration
10. Reabsorption
11. CFP
12. IFP
13. Filtration

EXERCISE 15 Stages of Tissue Healing

1. Inflammatory
2. Hemorrhage and inflammation; muscle spasm and pain; secondary edema formation; hematoma organization
3. Proliferative
4. Increased numbers of fibroblasts; decreased numbers of phagocytes; healing begins with the laying down of granulation tissues
5. Collagen remodeling based on demonstrated lines of stress on the tissue

Answers to Chapter 10 quiz

1. C body temperature, pH, and fluid balance
2. C erythrocyte
3. A leukocytes
4. D water
5. B thrombocytes
6. D hemostasis
7. B pulmonary and systemic
8. B It makes them more resilient and creates a recoil that is important for arterial flow.
9. D precapillary sphincter
10. C subclavian
11. D along the medial aspect of the lower extremity
12. A portal vein
13. A carotid artery

14. D acts as a protective covering that secretes serous fluid to decrease friction over the heart as it contracts
15. B pulmonary artery
16. C tricuspid
17. A left ventrical
18. D right atrium
19. B capillary fluid pressure
20. C blood pressure
21. B sinoatrial node
22. A skeletal muscle contraction
23. A acute
24. D Encourage pain-free movement throughout all stages.
25. D increased interstitial oncotic pressure

Chapter 11

EXERCISE 1 Lymphatic System Crossword

EXERCISE 2 The Lymphatic Vessels

1. Initial vessels
2. Subepidermis; blind-ended; anchor filaments
3. Dermis; epithelial; one-way valve
4. Initial vessels
5. Collectors
6. Subdermal; angions; smooth muscle
7. Pre-collectors
8. Trunks
9. Arteries; farther apart
10. Organ or body region
11. Ventral; cisterna chyli; thoracic duct
12. Subclavian; both lower

EXERCISE 3 Structure and Function of a Lymph Node

1. Lymphoid organs
2. Collectors
3. Lymph node beds
4. Catchments
5. Filters
6. Dust, pollen, and bacteria
7. Damaged cells and other cellular debris
8. Lymphocytes
9. Capsule
10. Trabeculae
11. Afferent lymph vessel
12. Nodule
13. Sinus
14. Efferent lymph vessel

EXERCISE 4 The Lymphatic Network

1. B Right lymphatic duct
2. H Axillary catchment
3. K Collector vessels
4. I Inguinal catchment
5. A Cisterna chyli
6. C Thoracic duct
7. J Internal jugular veins
8. B Right lymphatic duct
9. E Right subclavian vein
10. G Terminus of right lymphatic duct
11. C Thoracic duct
12. F Terminus of thoracic duct
13. D Left subclavian vein

EXERCISE 5 Edema Uptake Versus Lymphatic Flow

1. LF
2. LF
3. EU
4. EU
5. LF
6. EU
7. EU
8. LF
9. EU

EXERCISE 6 Mechanisms of Lymph Flow

1. Internal mechanisms
2. Siphon effect
3. Contraction of angions
4. Skeletal muscle contraction
5. Compression from adjacent arterial pulse
6. Respiratory pump

EXERCISE 7 Catchments and Watersheds

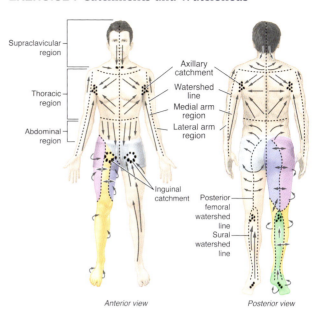

EXERCISE 8 Routes of Lymph Flow

Edema uptake @ anterior thigh:
1. H → 2. E → 3. F → 4. A → 5. C

Edema uptake @ right medial wrist:
1. K → 2. D → 3. B → 4. C

Edema uptake @ calf:
1. J → 2. G → 3. E → 4. F → 5. A → 6. C

Edema uptake @ right rib cage: 1. D → 2. B → 3. C

Edema uptake @ left lateral elbow:
1. L → 2. D → 3. C

Edema uptake @ anterior ankle:
1. I → 2. H → 3. E → 4. F → 5. A → 6. C

EXERCISE 9 Types of Edema

1. Edema caused by dysfunction or failure in the lymphatic system; congenital or genetic defect in lymphatic development
2. Weak or insufficient number of intralymphatic valves; low ratio of lymphatic vessels per cubic centimeter of tissue
3. Secondary lymphedema
4. Chemotherapy, radiation, infection, parasites (filarial)
5. Cardiovascular (dynamic) edema
6. Edema related to dysfunction or disease in the cardiovascular system; dynamic edema
7. Diabetes-related complications, venous insufficiency, or malnutrition
8. The localized and temporary swelling associated with soft tissue injury
9. Sprains, strains, hematomas

Answers to Chapter 11 quiz

1. A absorb fats from the digestive tract, return fluids and proteins to blood, and carry out several primary immune responses
2. C entwined in the interstitial spaces of the cardiovascular capillaries
3. D cells, proteins, foreign substances, and long-chain fatty acids
4. D gather fluid from multiple initial vessels and transport to the collectors
5. B a group of pre-collectors that connect different collectors for lymph transfer
6. C nonstructural pathways between cells called pre-lymphatic channels
7. B prevent backflow of fluid and divide the vessels into smaller segments
8. D terminus
9. D sagittal and umbilical
10. A 100%
11. B there must be negative pressure inside the lymphatic vessel network
12. B collecting well for lymph at the base of the thoracic duct
13. C initial capillaries
14. B respiratory pump and skeletal muscle contraction
15. D lymphotomes
16. A inguinal
17. C siphon effect and autonomic angion contraction
18. B lymphatic trunks
19. D dynamic edema
20. C lymphedema
21. A filters lymph of impurities and acts a primary site for immune responses
22. B thoracic
23. D just lateral to the clavicular head of the SCM and 2/3 subclavian
24. C This creates an internal pressure differential that facilitates filtration.
25. D lateral arm

Chapter 12

EXERCISE 1 Immunity Crossword

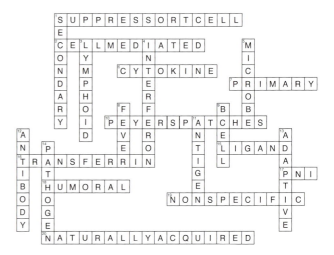

EXERCISE 2 Lymphoid Tissues

Note: Red type is used to designate the primary lymphoid tissues.

1. G red bone marrow
2. C lymph node
3. B spleen
4. D thymus
5. A tonsils
6. E Peyer's patches
7. H appendix
8. F adenoids

EXERCISE 3 Nonspecific Immune Defenses

1. Innate
2. Generic or universal
3. Any single type, or any specific kind

Chemical barriers—Chemicals that destroy or discourage the growth and/or spread of microbes, pathogens, and other foreign particles; include sebum, sweat, tears, gastric juice, saliva, urine, and vaginal secretions

Internal antimicrobial proteins—Proteins in the body such as interferons, complements, transferrins, and antimicrobial peptides that destroy microbes in a variety of ways

Phagocytes—Cells that eat microbes and cellular debris, such as neutrophils and macrophages

Natural killer cells—Roaming cells that kill infected body cells through cytolysis

Inflammation—Physiologic responses that fight and contain infectious agents by increasing vasodilation, capillary permeability, and phagocytosis; prepares tissue for repair

Fever—Elevated body temperature that speeds up metabolism to facilitate tissue repair; kills or inhibits the growth of certain bacteria; increases the effect of interferons

EXERCISE 4 Specific Immune Responses

Fill-in exercise:

1. Adaptive
2. Exposure
3. B and T
4. Specific
5. Antigen
6. Foreign particle or substance
7. Immune response

8. Antigen
9. Antigen receptor
10. B
11. Antibody-mediated
12. T
13. Cell-mediated

Diagram:

1. Pathogen
2. Antigen
3. APC
4. T cells
5. Cytotoxic T cells
6. Memory T cells
7. Helper T cells

8. Suppressor T cells
9. B cells
10. Plasma cells
11. Antibodies
12. Memory B cells
13. CMI
14. AMI

EXERCISE 6 Gaining Immunity

1. T
2. T
3. F
4. F

5. T
6. F
7. T
8. T

Answers to Chapter 12 quiz

1. C lymphocytes
2. D red bone marrow
3. B B cell
4. B pharyngeal
5. A acidity of gastric juices
6. A innate immune defenses
7. C Peyer's patches
8. A transferrins; complement proteins
9. B red bone marrow
10. B provide the first line of internal nonspecific defense
11. D epidermis of skin and mucous membranes
12. C chemotaxis
13. D plasma cells
14. C immunoglobulin
15. C vasodilation and phagocytosis
16. D tranferrins
17. B B lymphocytes

18. C It is an antigen-specific response and creates an immune memory.
19. A inhibit and stop the immune response process once the challenge has passed
20. B They are rendered ineffective.
21. D vaccinations
22. B a network of communication peptides called ligands
23. C humoral immunity
24. A cytotoxic T cells
25. D artificially acquired passive

Chapter 13

EXERCISE 1 Respiratory System Crossword

EXERCISE 2 Respiratory Structures

1. Frontal sinus
2. Nasal cavity
3. Oral cavity (mouth)
4. Pharynx
5. Larynx
6. Trachea
7. Bronchi

8. Bronchioles
9. Right lung
10. Left lung
11. Diaphragm
12. Bronchiole
13. Capillaries
14. Alveoli

EXERCISE 3 Matching Respiratory Organs

1. D pharynx
2. E nasal conchae
3. H sinuses
4. A trachea
5. K lungs
6. L alveoli

7. I bronchioles
8. F primary bronchi
9. G pleura
10. C larynx
11. J respiratory membrane
12. B respiratory cilia

EXERCISE 4 Upper or Lower Respiratory Tract

1. L
2. L
3. L
4. L
5. U
6. L
7. U
8. U
9. U
10. U

EXERCISE 5 Muscles of Ventilation

1. External intercostals, inhalation
2. Diaphragm, inhalation
3. Rectus abdominis, exhalation
4. Internal intercostals, exhalation
5. Scalenes, inhalation
6. Serratus anterior, inhalation
7. Pectoralis minor, inhalation
8. Sternocleidomastoid, inhalation

EXERCISE 6 Respiration

1. Oxygen and carbon dioxide exchange
2. Inside the lungs between the alveoli and the blood
3. In the capillary beds throughout the body between the blood and the interstitium
4. Exchange of gases between the alveoli and the blood
5. Internal respiration
6. Diffusion
7. Hemoglobin (Hb)
8. Plasma
9. Oxyhemoglobin (HbO$_2$)
10. Bicarbonate
11. Carbaminohemoglobin

EXERCISE 7 Respiration and Circulation

1. External respiration in the lungs
2. Internal respiration in the body tissues
3. Alveolus
4. Body cells
5. Pulmonary veins
6. Systemic arteries
7. Systemic veins
8. Pulmonary arteries

Arrows should show CO$_2$ moving out of and O$_2$ moving into the blood during external respiration.

Arrows should show CO$_2$ moving into and O$_2$ moving out of the blood during internal respiration.

Answers to Chapter 13 quiz

1. C help regulate temperature and fluid balance by eliminating heat and water
2. D alveoli
3. A prevent food from entering the trachea during swallowing
4. B warm and moisten air before it enters lungs
5. C trachea
6. C larynx
7. D trachea
8. A ventilation
9. C external respiration
10. D diffusion
11. C Carbon dioxide moves into the lungs and oxygen moves into the blood.
12. B increases in size
13. A diaphragm
14. C as oxyhemoglobin on red blood cells
15. D chemoreceptors and stretch receptors
16. D high blood levels of carbon dioxide
17. C inside the walls of the carotid and aortic arteries
18. B as bicarbonate ions
19. C internal respiration
20. A intercostal and phrenic

Chapter 14

EXERCISE 1 Digestive System Crossword

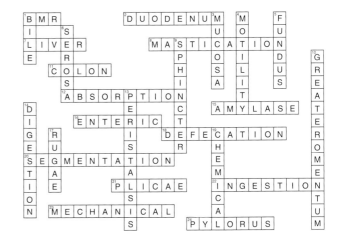

224   Answer Key

EXERCISE 2 Gastrointestinal Tract Versus Accessory Organs and Functions

1. GI
2. A
3. GI
4. GI
5. A
6. A
7. GI
8. A
9. GI
10. A
11. GI
12. GI
13. A

EXERCISE 3 Digestive System Organs

1. Salivary glands
2. Teeth
3. Tongue
4. Mouth (oral cavity)
5. Pharynx
6. Esophagus
7. Stomach
8. Liver
9. Gallbladder
10. Pancreas
11. Small intestine
12. Ascending colon
13. Transverse colon
14. Hepatic flexure
15. Splenic flexure
16. Descending colon
17. Sigmoid colon
18. Rectum
19. Anus
20. Duodenum
21. Jejunum
22. Ileum
23. Cecum
24. Appendix
25. Iliocecal valve

EXERCISE 4 Layers of the GI Tract

Matching:

1. G mucosa
2. J submucosa
3. I muscularis
4. B serosa
5. D myenteric plexus
6. F Peyer's patch
7. C mesentery
8. E submucosal plexus
9. H circular layer
10. A longitudinal layer

Diagram:

1. Mucosa
2. Peyer's patch (MALT)
3. Submucosal plexus
4. Submucosa
5. Longitudinal smooth muscle layer
6. Circular smooth muscle layer
7. Muscularis
8. Myenteric plexus
9. Serosa
10. Mesentery

EXERCISE 5 Functions of the Digestive System

1. Salivary amylase
2. Swallowing
3. Saliva
4. Peristalsis
5. Hydrochloric acid, pepsin
6. Pepsin
7. Peristalsis
8. Alcohol
9. Proteases, CCK
10. Mixing via segmentation
11. Segmentation, peristalsis
12. Glucose, triglycerides, amino acids
13. Mucus
14. Water

EXERCISE 6 Diagram the Functions of the GI Tract

1. Mouth (oral cavity)
2. Pharynx
3. Esophagus
4. Stomach
5. Small intestine
6. Large intestine
7. Anus

Ingestion: 1—eating

Mechanical digestion: 1—chewing; 4—churning; 5—segmentation for mixing

Chemical digestion: 1—amylase in the saliva; 4—gastric juices; 5—enzymes and bile from liver, gallbladder, and pancreas, plus enzymes produced by the SI

Motility: 1 and 2—swallowing; 3—peristalsis; 4—peristalsis/gastric emptying; 5—peristalsis; 6—peristalsis

Absorption: 1—sublingual medications, etc.; 4—medications and alcohol; 5—all nutrients; 6—water

Defecation: 7—elimination of feces

EXERCISE 7 Metabolism and Nutrients

1. Chemical reactions
2. Anabolic
3. Repaired
4. Synthesized
5. Catabolic
6. Produce ATP
7. Macronutrients
8. Glucose
9. Energy
10. Glycogen
11. Fat
12. Lipids
13. Glycerol; fatty acids
14. Adipose
15. Amino acids
16. Liver
17. Protein synthesis
18. Enzymes, receptors, antibodies, hormones, and/or ligands
19. Micronutrients
20. Serving as coenzymes in chemical reactions
21. Minerals
22. Blood; bone
23. Coenzymes that help regulate chemical reactions in the body (similar to vitamins)
24. Water

Answers to Chapter 14 quiz

1. A digestion
2. D defecation
3. C liver and gallbladder
4. B peritoneum
5. A mouth
6. C esophagus
7. B stomach
8. A salivary glands
9. D absorption of water
10. D ileocecal
11. B pancreas and duodenum
12. C insulate and cushion the abdominopelvic cavity
13. A splenic flexure
14. D regulation of digestive secretions and motility
15. D triglyceride
16. B absorb fats from the small intestine
17. C small intestine
18. A anabolism of amino acids
19. D secretin
20. C secretion of protein digestive enzymes

Chapter 15

EXERCISE 1 Urinary System Crossword

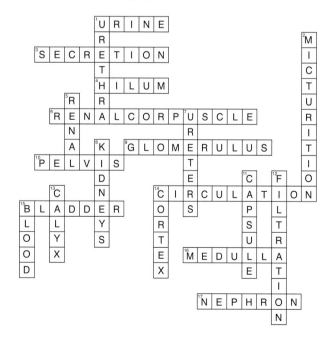

EXERCISE 2 Urinary System Organs

Diagram:

A. Urethra
B. Bladder
C. Ureters
D. Kidney
E. Diaphragm

Matching:

1. C
2. B
3. D
4. D
5. A
6. B
7. C
8. D
9. D
10. D

EXERCISE 3 Structure of the Kidneys

1. Renal cortex—Outer region of the kidney
2. Renal medulla—Inner region of the kidney
3. Renal capsule—Large fascial envelope that surrounds each kidney and attaches it to the abdominal wall
4. Renal pyramids—Triangle-shaped bundle of microscopic tubes within the renal medulla that collect urine from a specific group of nephrons
5. Nephron—Microscopic functional unit of the kidney
6. Calyx—Small cup at the bottom of a renal pyramid that collects urine and transfers it to the renal pelvis
7. Renal pelvis—Region of the kidney where urine is collected before being passed into the ureter

EXERCISE 4 Parts of a Nephron

1. Efferent arteriole
2. Glomerulus
3. Bowman's (glomerular) capsule
4. Afferent arteriole
5. Proximal convoluted tubule
6. Venule
7. Peritubular capillaries
8. Loop of Henle
9. Distal convoluted tubule
10. Collecting ducts

EXERCISE 5 Structure and Function of a Nephron

1. F glomerulus
2. J distal convoluted tubule
3. A filtration
4. B renal corpuscle
5. I collecting duct
6. C Bowman's capsule
7. H secretion
8. D proximal convoluted tubule
9. E reabsorption
10. G peritubular capillaries

EXERCISE 6 The Kidney's Role in Fluid Management

Your answers may vary, but might include the following:

Regulates blood pressure—directly related to managing fluid volume; decreased BP causes the release of aldosterone to support sodium retention and ADH to support water retention; increased BP increases urinary excretion

Regulates blood electrolytes—manages sodium ions, potassium ions, calcium ions, and phosphate ions

Regulates blood pH—balances levels of hydrogen ions, which determines acidity; balances bicarbonate ion levels, which influences blood alkalinity

Waste elimination—urea and ammonia from protein catabolism; uric acids from nucleic acid catabolism; bilirubin from RBC destruction; drugs; toxins; excess vitamins and minerals

Hormone production—calcitriol; erythropoietin

Answers to Chapter 15 quiz

1. D urethra, and ureters
2. A secretion of hormones
3. B bladder
4. D Ureters carry urine from kidneys to bladder and urethra goes from bladder to external environment.
5. B nephron
6. A renal cortex
7. B erythropoietin
8. D renal corpuscle
9. C pelvis
10. D Bowman's capsule and glomerulus
11. A renal corpuscle
12. B distal convoluted tubule
13. B reabsorption
14. A glomerulus
15. B micturition
16. C 95%
17. B uric acid
18. D at the more proximal end of the urethra
19. A external sphincter
20. D 97% to 99%

Chapter 16

EXERCISE 1 Reproductive System Crossword

EXERCISE 2 Mind Map of Common Characteristics

1, 2. M—testes; F—ovaries

3, 4. M—sperm; F—ova

5, 6. M—penis and scrotum; F—vulva

7, 8. M—seminal vesicles, epididymis, vas deferens, ejaculatory duct, urethra; F—fallopian tubes; uterus, vagina

9, 10. M—testosterone; F—estrogens, progesterone

11, 12. M—Leydig cells; F—follicles, corpus luteum

EXERCISE 3 Male Pelvic Anatomy

1. Bladder
2. Urethra
3. Penis
4. External urethral orifice
5. Testes
6. Scrotum
7. Epididymis
8. Vas deferens
9. Anus
10. Rectum
11. Bulbourethral gland
12. Prostate
13. Ejaculatory duct
14. Internal urethral orifice
15. Seminal vesicle

EXERCISE 4 Male Reproductive Structures and Functions

1. E seminal vesicle
2. I testes
3. G vas deferens
4. B seminiferous tubules
5. A epididymis
6. C ejaculatory duct
7. D Leydig cells
8. F prostate gland
9. H bulbourethral glands

Answer Key   227

EXERCISE 5 Female Pelvic Anatomy

1. Fallopian tube (oviduct)
2. Ovary
3. Bladder
4. Mons pubis
5. Clitoris
6. Urethra
7. Vaginal opening
8. Anus
9. Vagina
10. Rectum
11. Cervix
12. Uterus

EXERCISE 6 Female Reproductive Structures and Functions

1. H follicle
2. F corpus luteum
3. E endometrium
4. A fallopian tube
5. I fimbriae
6. D vagina
7. J uterus
8. B ovary
9. C placenta
10. G labia

Answers to Chapter 16 quiz

1. A gonads, accessory organs, genitalia, hormonal control processes
2. C expelling of an egg from the ovary
3. D prostate
4. B fertilization
5. D seminiferous tubules
6. C corpus luteum
7. A seminal vesicle
8. B vagina
9. C third week
10. C narrow distal zone
11. A progesterone
12. D secrete a milky fluid that prevents semen clotting
13. A inside the fallopian tube
14. C 1 through 5
15. D scrotum

The perfect tools for the times.

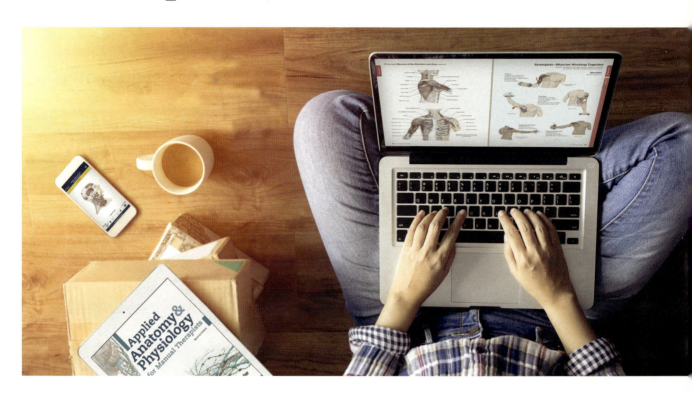

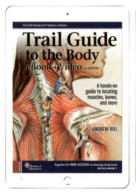 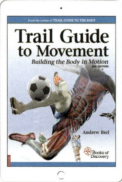 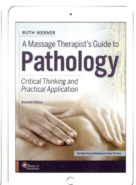 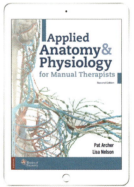

Discover our full suite of digital learning resources at
booksofdiscovery.com/GoDigital

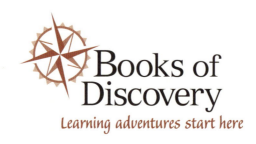

Learning adventures start here